ASPIRIN, PLATELETS AND STROKE

ASPIRIN, PLATELETS AND STROKE

Background for a Clinical Trial

Compiled and Edited by

WILLIAM S. FIELDS, M.D.

Professor of Neurology
The University of Texas Medical School
at Houston

and

WILLIAM K. HASS, M.D.

Professor of Neurology
New York University
School of Medicine

With 29 Contributors

WARREN H. GREEN, INC.
St. Louis, Missouri, U.S.A.

Published by

WARREN H. GREEN, INC.
10 South Brentwood Blvd.
St. Louis, Missouri 63105, U.S.A.

Library of Congress Catalog No. 74-153915

Printed in the United States of America

(190)

CONTRIBUTORS

Raymond B. Bauer, M.D. *Professor of Neurology, Wayne State University, Detroit, Michigan.*

William P. Blackmore, M.D., Ph.D., *Director, Clinical Pharmacology, Sterling Winthrop Research Institute, Rensselaer, New York.*

Norman E. Chase, M.D., *Professor of Radiology, New York University Medical Center, New York, New York.*

Mark L. Dyken, M.D., *Professor of Neurology, Indiana University School of Medicine, Indianapolis, Indiana.*

William K. Ehrenfeld, M.D., *Associate Professor of Surgery (Vascular), University of California Medical Center, San Francisco, California.*

Geoffrey Evans, M.B., *Associate Professor of Surgery, McMaster University, Hamilton, Ontario, Canada.*

William S. Fields, M.D., *Professor of Neurology, The University of Texas Medical School at Houston, Houston, Texas.*

Anthony P. Fletcher, M.D., *Associate Professor of Medicine, Washington University School of Medicine, St. Louis, Missouri.*

Ralph Frankowski, Ph.D., *Assistant Professor of Biometry. The University of Texas School of Public Health at Houston, Houston, Texas.*

William K. Hass, M.D., *Professor of Neurology, New York University Medical Center, New York, New York.*

Richard Janeway, M.D., *Associate Professor of Neurology, The Bowman Gray School of Medicine of Wake Forest University, Winston-Salem, North Carolina.*

Thomas G. Kantor, M.D., *Associate Professor of Clinical Medicine, New York University Medical Center, New York, New York.*

Pulla R. S. Kishore, M.D., *Instructor in Radiology, New York University Medical Center, New York, New York.*

Irvin I. Kricheff, M.D., *Professor of Radiology, New York University Medical Center, New York, New York.*

Ben Marr Lanman, M.D., *Medical Director, Bristol-Myers Company, New York, New York.*

Aaron J. Marcus, M.D., *Associate Professor of Medicine, Cornell University Medical School, New York, New York.*

Holt A. McDowell, Jr., M.D., *Associate Professor of Surgery, The University of Alabama School of Medicine, Birmingham, Alabama.*

Clark H. Millikan, M.D., *Professor of Neurology, Mayo Graduate School of Medicine, Mayo Clinic, Rochester, Minnesota.*

Wesley S. Moore, M.D., *Assistant Professor of Surgery, University of California School of Medicine, and Chief, Vascular Surgery, Veterans Administration Hospital, San Francisco, California.*

James F. Mustard, M.D., *Professor of Pathology, McMaster University, Hamilton, Ontario, Canada.*

Marian A. Packham, Ph.D., *Visiting Professor, Department of Pathology, McMaster University, Hamilton, Ontario, Canada.*

Sidney Riegelman, Ph.D., *Pharmacokinetic Research Labs, University of California School of Pharmacy, San Francisco, California.*

Mervyn A. Sahud, M.D., *Research Associate, Department of Medicine, University of California School of Medicine, San Francisco, California.*

Reuel A. Stallones, M.D., M.P.H., *Dean, The University of Texas School of Public Health at Houston, Houston, Texas.*

H. Grant Taylor, M.D., *Dean, The University of Texas Graduate School of Biomedical Sciences, Division of Continuing Education, Houston, Texas.*

Edward B. Truitt, Ph.D., *Senior Research Fellow in Pharmacology, Battelle Memorial Institute, Columbus, Ohio.*

Harvey J. Weiss, M.D., *Associate Clinical Professor of Medicine, Columbia University College of Physicians and Surgeons, New York, New York.*

Frank Yatsu, M.D., *Chief, Neurology Service, University of California San Francisco General Hospital, San Francisco, California.*

Marjorie B. Zucker, Ph.D., *Associate Professor of Pathology, New York University Medical Center, New York, New York.*

PREFACE

From the time of Hippocrates, when the bark of the willow tree was recommended for the relief of the discomfort and pain of childbirth, there has been an increasing therapeutic use of the salicylates to ease pain (1). "Among the many useful discoveries which this age hath made, there are very few which better deserve the attention of the public than what I am going to lay before you," thus wrote Edward Stone in part to the president of the Royal Society in 1763, describing his experience with the bark of the willow tree (2). Although it is impossible to accurately appraise, it is highly probable that the salicylates have played the major role in reducing the aggregate of pain and suffering in the civilized communities of the world.

It was not until sixty-five years later that the active ingredient, salicin, was isolated from the bark of the willow tree. In 1953, Charles Frederick von Gerhardt reported the successful preparation of the acetic acid ester of salicylic acid (aspirin), but this accomplishment also remained unnoticed for another fifty years.

In the meantime, Lister's successful use of carbolic acid for its disinfecting qualities stimulated a German physician to search for a way in which carbolic acid could be given internally with safety. In 1870, he placed the problem before Hermann Klobe, professor of chemistry at the University of Leipsig. Professor Klobe was the right man. Twenty years previously he had synthesized salicylic acid from carbolic acid and recalled that his synthesized product slowly broke down and became carbolic acid. He reasoned that salicylic acid would similarly convert to carbolic acid in the body and thus become the "germ killing" successor to Lister's carbolic

---

1. Gross, Martin, and Greenberg, Leon: *The Salicylates.* Hillhouse Press, New Haven, Conn.
2. Stone, E.: An Account of the Success of the Bark of the Willow in the Cure of Agues. *Philosophical Transactions, 53:*195, 1763.

acid. Accordingly in 1874 the new "germ killer," salicylic acid, was announced (3). Doctors clamored for the new product. It was applied topically and administered internally for many kinds of diseases. It was even used as a food preservative. Within a year, however, reports indicated that while salicylic acid seemingly made patients feel better, the drug did not effect cure. It would reduce fever and relieve pain but otherwise did not seem to alter the course of disease.

Hermann Klobe's "germ killer" theory was thus disproved, but salicylic acid did reduce fever and relieve pain and in particular did reduce fever, pain and swollen joints of the rheumatic. It was also reported to be useful for those suffering with headaches, neuralgia, and neuritis. Professor Kolbe had found an effective, economical antipyretic and analgesic. To meet the widespread demands for the product, other pharmaceutical companies became interested and assigned their chemists the task of producing the compound.

At Friedrich Bayer and Company in Germany, Felix Hoffman, a young staff chemist whose father was ill with rheumatoid arthritis, searched the literature and found the compound discarded by von Gerhardt. The drug had remained in obscurity for forty-six years until Hoffman and Arthur Eichengrun brought it to clinical trial and ultimately a successful clinical evaluation. From the memoirs of Eichengrun, written in a Nazi concentration camp and published in *Die Pharmazie* in 1950 comes the story of the rejection of aspirin by the scientific director of Bayer's, Dr. Heinrick Dreser, and Eichengrun's collaboration with Hoffman forcing a reassessment of the compounds potential usefulness. Hoffman's father was one of the first to receive the drug.

An extensive bibliography on aspirin exists wherein the chemistry, pharmacology and toxicology are well covered as are many of the therapeutic uses of aspirin. There is still, nevertheless, much to be learned about the mechanism of action of the compound. The answers to "how" aspirin relieves pain and reduces temperatures will be determined. These answers may reveal still more applications for this safe and inexpensive drug whose contribution in allevating the pain and physical discomfitures of society is unexceeded by any other known compound.

---

3. Huchwalt, Carroll A. *Pharmacy International*, pg. 16, February 1957.

It is interesting that even one of the adverse reactions of this compound, usually attributed to over-dosage with aspirin, is the subject of this monograph wherein the possible use of aspirin as an anticoagulant for the prevention of stroke will be explored.

— H. Grant Taylor

ACKNOWLEDGMENTS

The editors wish to acknowledge the financial support provided by the following pharmaceutical firms:

Bristol-Myers Products
Norwich Pharmacal Company
Sterling Drug, Inc.

Without this assistance, it would not have been possible to bring together this group of clinicians and laboratory scientists to discuss a possible solution to a common health problem of extreme importance.

* * *

The support of the staff of The University of Texas Graduate School of Biomedical Sciences, Division of Continuing Education, is gratefully acknowledged. Our sincere appreciation is also extended to the administration and staff of St. Anthony Center for providing the facilities for the conference.

* * *

The editors also wish to express appreciation to Mrs. Jane Lester and Mrs. Verna McCarthy for their assistance in preparing and editing the final manuscript for publication.

W.S.F.
W.K.H.

CONTENTS

PART III
PHARMACOLOGY OF SALICYLATES

PART IV
CONTROLLED CLINICAL TRIALS

ASPIRIN, PLATELETS AND STROKE

PART I

TRANSIENT CEREBRAL ISCHEMIC ATTACKS

Moderators

William S. Fields, M.D.
William K. Hass, M.D.

Chapter I

INTRODUCTION

WILLIAM S. FIELDS, M.D.

In the prevention of arterial thrombosis and embolism, interest is currently being focused on certain drugs (aspirin among others) which are capable of inhibiting platelet aggregation. In the final analysis, any potential worth of these drugs must be proven in a major clinical trial wherein their effect on recurrence of ischemic events or mortality rate from cerebral infarction or myocardial infarction is evaluated.

It is our sincere hope that the formal presentations during this conference, and the discussions which follow, will provide background material for planning a controlled clinical trial in which several investigators may desire participation, and from which there may be answers to questions which are at present still unanswered.

Some of the persons present at this conference have been participants in a cooperative study supported by the National Heart and Lung Institute over the past ten years. This study, known officially as the Joint Study of Extracranial Arterial Occlusion, has a Central Registry for the acquisition, storage and analysis of information collected at the cooperating and participating centers in this country and South America. The Central Registry is operated under the auspices of The University of Texas Medical School at Houston.

The initial objective of this joint study was to determine the role of arterial reconstructive surgery in the management of stroke. Fortunately, there have been a number of additional by-products, not the least of which was the demonstration of the value of so-called "four-vessel arteriography" in the diagnosis and management of occlusive cerebrovascular disease and the opportunity to learn more about the demography of a stroke population. This kind of study provides only very limited information about the natural history of stroke, but it does yield considerable data regarding the clinical course of persons who are already symptomatic of cerebrovascular disease.

At the time this study was first planned and then undertaken, it was considered by most of the participants that the significance of a lesion in the extracranial arteries was determined by the degree and length of a stenosis within the lumen of one or more of the principal vessels leading to the brain. These lesions were supposed to be responsible for alterations in blood pressure and blood flow within the more distal branches. Even at that time, however, some clinicians suggested that thromboembolism had a very distinct role in the production of some transient cerebral ischemic attacks. For this reason, a controlled trial of anticoagulant therapy was undertaken in the early 1960's but, unfortunately, the conclusions of this trial were not too widely accepted. Furthermore, this study suffered from one very distinct disadvantage, namely, that the anatomical description of the lesion was not possible because arteriography was not a prerequisite for the admission of subjects.

Within two years of the outset of the controlled trial of surgery in extracranial arterial occlusion, it became obvious that treatment comparisons would not be meaningful unless the subjects were randomly allocated into two groups in accordance with a predetermined statistical design. One group would be operated, and the other one unoperated. They would then be followed for like periods of time.

In the planning of this aspect of the study, which has been referred to as the "randomized clinical trial," the ground rules for the admission of subjects were drawn up in 1961, at a time when our knowledge was still somewhat meager. As a consequence, the degree of stenosis was considered to be the most significant factor, and lesions which were non-obstructing, yet which might give rise to platelet or fibrin emboli, were not considered.

This is frequently one of the pitfalls in an experimental design for a controlled clinical trial, since the investigators become locked into certain decisions which remain unaltered or unalterable during the course of the trial. In the aforementioned study, which is now in its closing phase, the selection of candidates for the trial, in which subjects were randomly allocated to surgery or no surgery, was by criteria which would no longer be considered adequate. Only those subjects were admitted to the trial whose lesions were demonstrated radiographically to obstruct the lumen of a major artery to an extent greater than 30%, when estimated in x-ray films taken in two planes. This, of course, made it imperative that careful biplane angiographic studies be done in order to properly delineate the lesion and make possible this type of measurement.

Several years after the decision was made to include only subjects with 30% or greater stenosis, the investigators came to recognize that there were individuals who were symptomatic and whose symptoms could not be distinguished from the others, and in whom no lesions were demonstrated arteriographically, at least by the techniques that we had available to us at that time. Later, however, we began to appreciate that there were ulcerated lesions within the artery which could be seen in the x-ray films, although these lesions were not obstructive. Unfortunately these patients were not admissible to the controlled clinical trial under the ground rules established at the outset.

This kind of experience should provide us with a lesson which will enable us to establish another clinical trial with a more appropriate design. A flexible design could be altered, even when the trial is underway, in such a manner that it would not influence the value of the information retrieved.

The benefit of carotid endarterectomy in the treatment of obstructing extracranial carotid artery lesions has become well established and has met with fairly wide acceptance. It seems reasonable, however, to consider a cooperative study in which patients with the hemispheric type of transient cerebral ischemic attacks or attacks of monocular blindness could be admitted to a controlled clinical trial in which there would be a comparison of a specific medical therapy and carotid surgery.

It has been suggested that the medical therapy be in the form of aspirin, which has been shown *in vitro* to produce marked inhibition of collagen-induced platelet aggregation and the subsequent platelet release reaction. Furthermore, animal experiments have clearly demonstrated a reduction in intra-arterial clotting following the administration of aspirin in comparatively small doses.

Aspirin is a widely used, non-prescription drug of which the dosage we propose to use is considered non-toxic. The occasional case of allergy or other specific idiosyncrasy to the drug is really insignificant when one considers the number of persons who take aspirin regularly, for either headache or rheumatic pain, in doses considerably larger than those proposed for this investigation. Every precaution must be taken, however, to exclude these cases from such a clinical trial.

Chapter II

THE ISCHEMIC STROKE SYNDROME: A NEUROLOGIST'S VIEW

WILLIAM K. HASS, M.D.

To almost all laymen and many physicians, the word "stroke" conjures up visions of a bedridden hemiplegic, often unable to speak, or at best an elderly individual with a completed stroke, shuffling about with a cane, the days of his creativity and social contribution to an end. Volumes have been devoted to supportive therapy in the acute stage and rehabilitation therapy of the completed stroke.

To many neurologists who have felt impotent in the face of the permanent brain damage which underlies the completed stroke, both from the vascular surgical and medical standpoint, it has become apparent that the time to treat the common ischemic stroke is when it threatens, or even before. If such essentially prophylactic long-term treatment could be swiftly and safely accomplished in an ischemic stroke-prone individual, this would be a matter of no little importance.

Obviously, what I have said of ischemic stroke also applies to ischemic heart disease. Lacking means of specific prevention of atherosclerosis, the common underlying etiologic mechanism, it becomes necessary to take a new hard look at the process of cerebral ischemia, and to ask why atherosclerosis causes cerebral symptoms in some and not in others who have an apparently equal if not greater measure of extra- or intracranial arterial stenosis or occlusion.

The disease we are discussing is exceedingly common. About three-quarters of all patients with transient and persistant focal cerebral dysfunction of rapid onset suffer from cerebral ischemia. The average age of that portion of the patient population which presents at a hospital with cerebral ischemia is sixty-one (1). Cerebral ischemia, therefore, is not just a disorder of advanced senescence but very much a disease afflicting many people who are still in their active, creative years.

Prospective angiographic studies in symptomatic patients with transient or persistent ischemic stroke syndromes have revealed that more than two-thirds have atherosclerotic or atherothrombotic lesions, or both, which occupy 30% or more of the lumen at a surgically accessible portion of the extracranial arterial tree (2). Only 7% of patients have lesions which are confined to the intracranial vessels. Forty percent of all right and 40% of all left cervical carotid arteries in this population, when examined by angiography, exhibited significant stenosis or occlusion. The internal carotid arteries, most often at or near the bifurcation, are involved by a stenotic or occlusive process ten times more frequently than the middle cerebral arteries. Recent post-mortem studies have banished the old notion that middle cerebral arterial disease is a frequent occurrence, and established the rarity of primary *in situ* atherosclerotic lesions of the middle cerebral artery in comparison with the frequent occurrence of primary lesions in the carotid arteries of the neck (3).

The 1961 Mayo study of autopsies on 100 patients over fifty, *not* preselected for cerebral ischemic symptoms, revealed forty cases with 50% or greater stenosis of at least one major extracranial artery or aortic ostium (4). Every case, however, showed some degree of degenerative arteriosclerosis in at least one extracranial artery. Only eleven cases showed one or more vessels with frank occlusion.

The incidence in this series of carotid luminal stenosis of 25% or greater, as in subsequent post-mortem and angiographic studies, was much greater than the incidence of vertebral lesions of similar magnitude. However, only 16 of the 40 patients with significant arterial lesions of 50% stenosis or greater demonstrated frank cerebral infarction on brain examination (only 33 brain autopsies). A cerebral infarct was also found in three of 60 patients (52 brain autopsies) with minimal arteriosclerosis of the cervical arteries. This is a much smaller percentage, but is nevertheless a thought-provoking observation, since the maximal degree of cervical arterial compromise exceeded that in the intracranial arteries in 93% of the patients.

We observe, therefore, that one may find some patients having infarction without frank arterial occlusion or even what we used to call "significant" atherosclerotic or atherothrombotic lesions, and, on the other hand, patients with high grade stenotic or frank occlusive arterial lesions who do not suffer cerebral infarction. Thus, the first paradox: infarction without apparent arterial occlusion, and arterial occlusion without infarction.

Formerly it had been customary to explain attacks of focal cerebral ischemia occurring distal to frank carotid occlusion by invoking the mechanism of systemic hypotension and secondary collateral arterial failure (5). That such a mechanism only rarely obtains has been clear from my own experience and cases cited by others (6). Further, Francis Murphey has told many of us that only one of his 150 patients with ligated carotid arteries for aneurysm has developed a *tardy* hemiparesis in the territory of the ligated vessel after a 5 to 27 year follow-up (7).

Thus, we have a second paradox: a patient may experience long-term freedom from cerebral symptoms, in spite of complete spontaneous or iatrogenic *occlusion* of a carotid artery; whereas, the great majority of patients who present with symptoms of transient or persistent cerebral ischemia exhibit arterial *stenosis* rather than occlusion.

If one follows atherosclerotic lesions by a series of arteriographic studies, as the Wayne group did, one finds that the majority of the atherosclerotic lesions remain stable, while a small but significant number of lesions show sharp and significant changes, sometimes quite suddenly, in the atherosclerotic plaques (8). Consequently, atherosclerotic plaques may be for years a benign, though perhaps conspicuous feature, of the vascular landscape and then change quite suddenly. It is this dynamic transformation which probably underlies sudden changes in cerebral function and, as many of us feel, provides an explanation of the pathogenesis of cerebral ischemic events. Fresh atherothrombotic change in carotid plaques with arterial-arterial embolism now appears to play a major role in the pathogenesis of cerebral ischemia, as was suggested by four of Fisher's early cases (9), and documented in the carefully detailed cases of Gunning, Pickering, Robb-Smith and Ross Russell (10).

Dr. Kricheff will show us that certain specific alterations in plaques, particularly those in the cervical carotid arteries, are the significant angiographic features of the ischemic syndrome (11). He will point out that these lesions begin with irregularities of the intimal surface, progress to ulceration, and contribute to the propagation of small arterial-arterial emboli into the distal distribution of the middle cerebral artery. Dr. Moore will undoubtedly show that ulceration in carotid plaques may occur not only in the presence of high-grade stenosis, but also in carotid arteries where the lumina are minimally compromised by the atherosclerotic process (12).

Our discussions here, therefore, will consider a process which begins as platelet agglutination on an ulcerated extracranial arterial plaque. This may lead to deposition of friable fibrinoplatelet material, which may embolize into the distal portion of the carotid arterial tree. When embolization occurs into the arterioles of the ocular fundus, fibrinoplatelet material may be seen as "white lines" moving slowly, then rapidly, through these vessels (13). Initially, when a plaque breaks down, emboli representing cholesterol fragments can be observed in the retinal arteries. These were originally described by Hollenhorst as "bright plaques" (14, 15).

There is, therefore, much evidence to support our present hypothesis that ulcerative changes in a plaque, along with secondary platelet aggregation and subsequent arterial-arterial embolization and/or occlusive thrombosis, is the usual but by no means exclusive pathogenic mechanism in many patients with ischemic stroke syndromes. This new view resolves, in part at least, the paradoxes which I have cited. As a result, neurologists are now turning to therapeutic agents which will modify these events.

In selected cases, surgical excision of a segmental stenotic carotid plaque has certainly proved effective in diminishing the frequency of recurrent transient cerebral ischemic episodes and frank completed stroke in the territory of the operated carotid artery. Surgery is not without risk, but, where operative mortality and morbidity can be kept below 2%, surgery will continue to be a mode of prophylactic therapy favored by many for ischemic stroke syndromes (16, 17).

Pending final results of the controlled clinical trial of

extra-cranial arterial surgery for stroke, many clinicians have waited on the sidelines for a concept of the pathogenesis of ischemic stroke which would point to a rational *medical* therapy. Some of these physicians have employed anticoagulants in the management of recurrent transient ischemic attacks, often with temporary success. They treat, however, in the face of the ever-present danger of lethal hemorrhagic complications (18, 19). To some of us, a more safe and rational prophylactic therapy would prevent platelet aggregation on an ulcerated plaque and, therefore, prevent the development of friable fibrinoplatelet material or frank thrombus in an artery. An agent which would accomplish this would provide us with a much more desirable form of medical therapy.

The recent studies of aspirin as an inhibitor of collagen-induced platelet agglutination (20, 21) and the exciting new results that Dr. Evans will present from his pilot study, have prompted us to convene this meeting. A talented group from many medical specialities will examine the available data and consider the establishment of a cooperative study of aspirin and other platelet anti-aggregants in the prophylactic treatment of the ischemic stroke syndrome.

REFERENCES

1. Fields, W.S., North, R.R., Hass, W.K., Galbraith, S.G., Wylie, E.J., Ratinov, G., Burns, M.N., Macdonald, M.C., and Meyer, J.S.: Joint study of extracranial arterial occlusion as a cause of stroke. I. Organization of study and survey of patient population. *JAMA*, *203*:961-968, 1968.
2. Hass, W.K., Fields, W.S., North, R.R., Kricheff, I.I., Chase, N.E., and Bauer, R.B.: Joint study of extracranial arterial occlusion. II. Arteriography, techniques, sites, and complication. *JAMA*, *203*:955-960, 1968.
3. Lhermitte, F., Gautier, S.C., and Derouesne, C.: Nature of occlusions of the middle cerebral artery. *Neurology*, *20*:82-88, 1970.
4. Martin, M.J., Whisnant, J.P., and Sayre, G.P.: Occlusive vascular disease of the extracranial cerebral circulation. *Arch. Neurol.*, *3*:530-538, 1961.
5. Rothenberg, S.F. and Corday, E.: Etiology of the transient cerebral stroke. *JAMA*, *164*:2005, 1957.
6. Kendell, R.E. and Marshall, J.: Role of hypotension in the genesis of transient focal cerebral ischemic attacks. *Brit. Med. J.*, *2*:344-348, 1963.
7. Murphey, F.: *In Cerebral Vascular Diseases, Fourth Conference.* Millikan, C.H., Siekert, R.G., and Whisnant, J.P. (eds.) New York, Grune and Stratton, 1965, p. 196.

8. Bauer, R.B., Boulos, R.S., and Meyer, J.S.: Natural history and surgical treatment of occlusive cerebrovascular disease evaluated by serial arteriography. *Am. J. Roent.*, *104*:1-17, 1968.
9. Fisher, C.M.: Occlusion of the carotid artery: further experiences. *Arch. Neurol. and Psychiat.*, *72*:187-204, 1954.
10. Gunning, A.J., Pickering, G.W., Robb-Smith, A.H.T., and Ross Russell, R.: Mural thrombosis of the internal carotid artery and subsequent embolism. *Quart. J. Med.*, *33*:155-195, 1964.
11. Ring, A.B.: *The Neglected Cause of Stroke.* St. Louis, Mo., Warren H. Green, Inc., Dec. 1969, pp. 1-214.
12. Moore, W.S. and Hall, A.D.: Ulcerated atheroma of the carotid artery, a cause of transient cerebral ischemia. *Am. J. Surg.*, *116*:237-242, 1968.
13. Fisher, C.M.: Observations of the fundus oculi in transient monocular blindness. *Neurology*, *9*:333-347, 1959.
14. Hollenhorst, R.W.: Significance of bright plaques in the retinal arterioles. *Trans. Amer. Ophthol. Soc.*, *59*:252-273, 1966.
15. David, N.J., Klintworth, G.K., Friedberg, S.S., and Dillon, M.: Fatal atheromatous cerebral embolism associated with bright plaques in the retinal arterioles. *Neurology*, *13*:708-713, 1963.
16. Fields, W.S., Maslenikov, V., Meyer, J.S., Hass, W.K., Remington, R.D., and Macdonald, M.: Joint Study of Extracranial Arterial Occlusion. V. Prognosis in operated and non-operated patients with transient cerebral ischemic attacks. *JAMA*, *211*:1993-2003, 1970.
17. Thompson, J.E.: *Surgery for Cerebrovascular Insufficiency (Stroke).* Springfield, Ill., Charles C. Thomas, 1968, pp. 1-96.
18. Fisher, C.M.: Anticoagulant therapy in cerebral thrombosis and cerebral embolism. A national co-operative study, interim report. *Neurology*, *11* (No. 4, Part 2): 119-131, 1961.
19. Baker, R.N.: An evaluation of anticoagulant therapy in the treatment of cerebrovascular disease. Report of the Veterans Administration Co-operative Study of atherosclerosis, neurology section. *Neurology*, *11* (No. 4, Part 2): 132-138, 1961.
20. Weiss, H.J., Aledort, L.M., and Kochwa, S.: The effect of salicylates on the hemostatic properties of platelets in man. *J. Clin. Invest.*, *47*:2169-2180, 1968.
21. Evans, G., Packham, M.A., Nishizawa, E.E., Mustard, J.F., and Murphy, E.A.: The effect of acetylsalicylic acid on platelet function. *J. Exp. Med.*, *128*:877-894, 1968.

Chapter III

ULCERATED ATHEROMA OF CAROTID ARTERY AND CEREBRAL EMBOLISM*

PULLA R. S. KISHORE, M.D., NORMAN E. CHASE, M.D., and IRVIN I. KRICHEFF, M.D.

For the past few years, atherosclerotic lesions at the bifurcation of the extracranial carotid arteries have been recognized as a source of the embolization resulting in transient cerebral ischemic episodes. Ulceration of atheromatous carotid plaques is felt to increase the incidence of embolization, and there have been reports in the literature of relief from intermittent ischemic episodes following endarterectomy (1, 2). However, until now, no correlative study has been made comparing the presence of ulcerative plaques and embolic occlusion of middle cerebral branches demonstrated by angiography.

The purpose of this investigation was first to evaluate the 1). incidence of ulcerated atheromata at the bifurcation of the extracranial carotid arteries and other aorto-cranial vessels in patients with cerebrovascular disease, and 2) to compare the incidence of middle cerebral branch occlusions in these patients relative to the arteriosclerotic status of the carotid arteries.

MATERIAL AND METHOD

The incidence of ulcerated plaques in the carotid arteries and the aorto-cranial vessels of the vertebro-basilar system was investigated by examining the angiograms of 133 carotid arteries and 130 subclavian vertebro-basilar systems in 71 randomly selected patients studied for cerebrovascular insufficiency as part of the

*Supported in part by NINDS Neuroradiology Training Grant No. NBO 5433-05.

cooperative stroke study. No attempt was made either to select or evaluate these patients on the basis of their clinical status.

The incidence of middle cerebral branch occlusions relative to extracranial carotid artery status was evaluated in 82 patients. To the original 71, we added 11 patients with angiographic evidence of ulcerated carotid plaques who were investigated in our department during the period of time this work was in progress. These patients were included in the study on the basis of the presence of an ulcerated plaque without regard to intracranial vascular status. Biostatistical consultation assured us of the validity of including this material.

Patients were studied by right and left percutaneous retrograde brachial angiography and left common carotid angiography. No aortic arch studies were performed.

All the angiograms were evaluated without knowledge of the clinical history of the patient except that the patients had been admitted to the stroke study for evaluation of cerebrovascular disease. Surgical anatomic findings were not known and were obtained later in 31 of 34 patients who underwent surgery. The status of the extracranial vasculature was described as either normal, smooth stenosis, irregular stenosis, ulcerated plaque, or complete occlusion.

A lesion was considered to be an ulcerated plaque when a definite collection of contrast material was seen giving a crater-like appearance. These ulcers appear as a positive contrast shadow in a negative atheroma narrowing the carotid artery and they are usually seen on the posterior wall. The anterior oblique views so often obtained in aortic arch studies will miss most ulcers, for it is necessary to see the plaque in tangential projections. The lateral view is generally the best, and then ulcers are easily seen (Fig. 1).

Occasionally, ulcers may be more difficult to diagnose. They may be quite smooth, they may masquerade as a curve in the vessel, or as a normal area between two stenotic plaques. However, if the artery is studied on serial films, one will note that with an ulcer the contrast material will remain within the niche for a longer period of time than it will in the general arterial lumen (Figs. 2A & 2B). Though this is probably due in part to the dependent position of most ulcers, it should be noted that this delay in emptying does not occur with curves or in normal areas

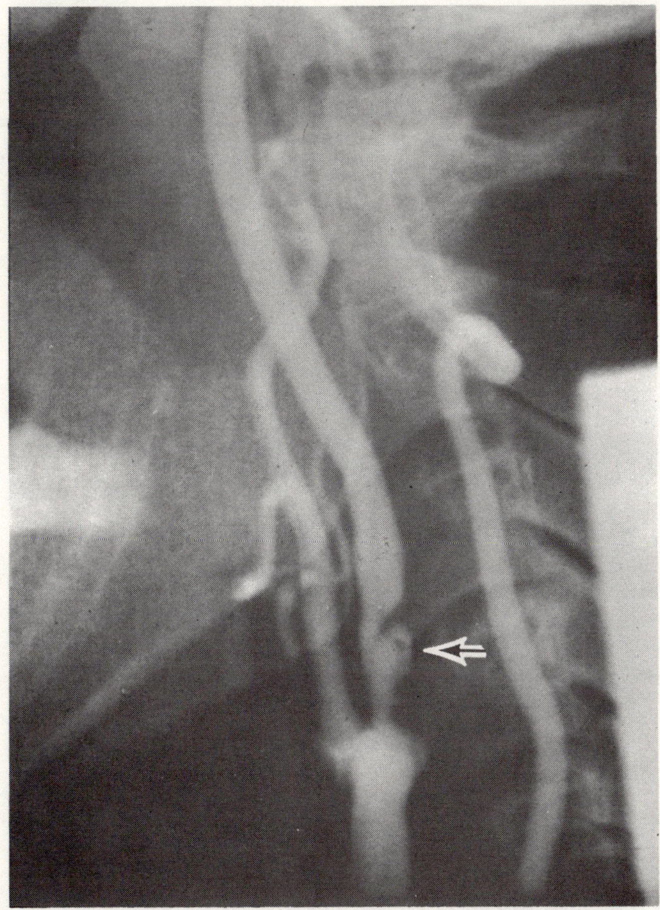

Figure 1. Right brachial angiogram on lateral view of the skull showing an ulcer *(arrow)* in the atheromatous plaque in the right internal carotid artery at origin.

between two stenotic plaques. The term "irregular stenosis" was used when a definite ulceration was not seen, but the arterial lumen was narrowed by a rough-surfaced plaque (Fig. 3).

Middle cerebral branch occlusions were diagnosed by evidence of 1) stasis in a vessel shown by delayed filling or delayed emptying; 2) collateral circulation; 3) capillary blush, or 4) an absent branch (3,4).

Though most branch occlusions are felt to be embolic, the

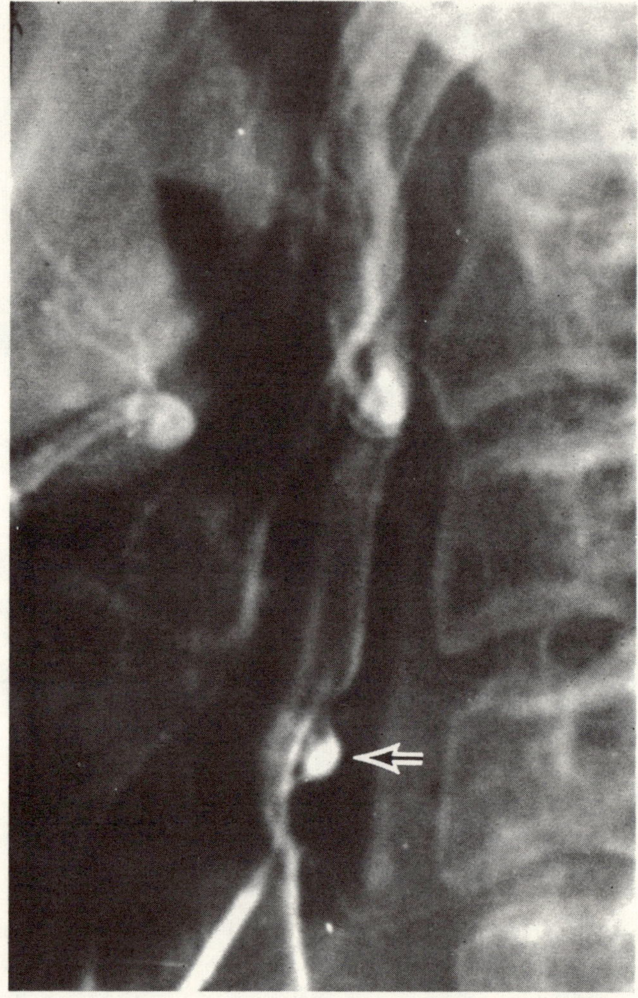

Figure 2A. Left common carotid angiogram on lateral view 2 seconds after the injection showing the contrast material in ulcer crater *(arrow)*. Note the disappearance of contrast material in the rest of the artery.

actual angiographic distinction between embolus and local arteriosclerotic occlusion may be difficult or impossible. A diagnosis of embolic occlusion can be made with certainty only when a well-defined convex filling defect is seen at the branching of a vessel (Fig. 4). Migration or dissolution of an obstruction as seen on serial films or on a subsequent angiographic study is also

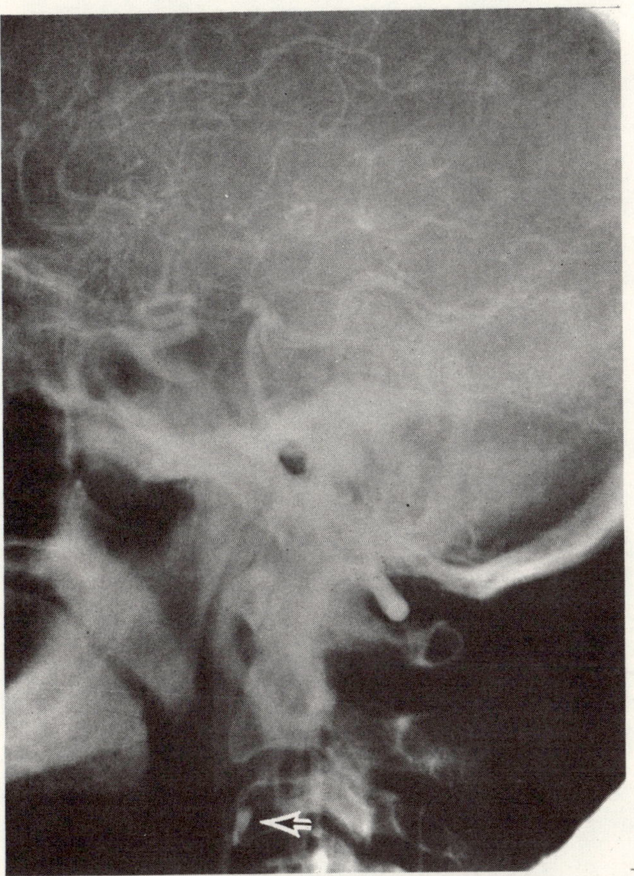

Figure 2B. Right brachial angiogram on lateral view of skull showing retention of contrast material in the ulcer crater *(arrow)* of internal carotid artery at the end of 3 seconds after injection.

diagnostic of an embolic occlusion. In cases where embolus blocks the vessel completely or is incorporated into the wall of the vessel projecting into or narrowing the lumen, the angiographic differentiation between embolic occlusion and local occlusion is difficult or impossible. The presence of generalized vascular disease involving multiple intracranial or extracranial branches probably makes the diagnosis of embolic occlusion less likely.

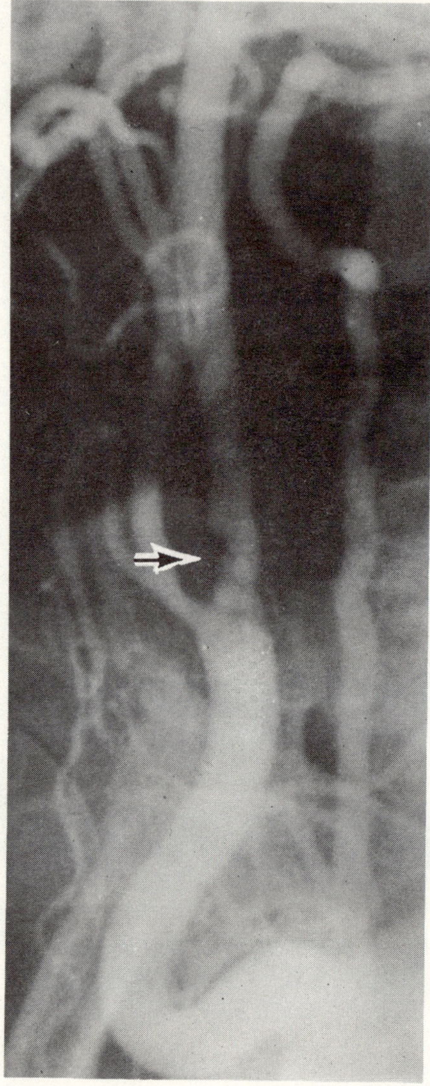

Figure 3. Right brachial angiogram on lateral oblique view of chest showing irregular plaque *(arrow)* at the origin of internal carotid artery. No ulcer is demonstrated.

RESULTS

Five ulcerated plaques were seen in the vertebrobasilar system on 130 brachial angiograms performed in 71 patients. This is the

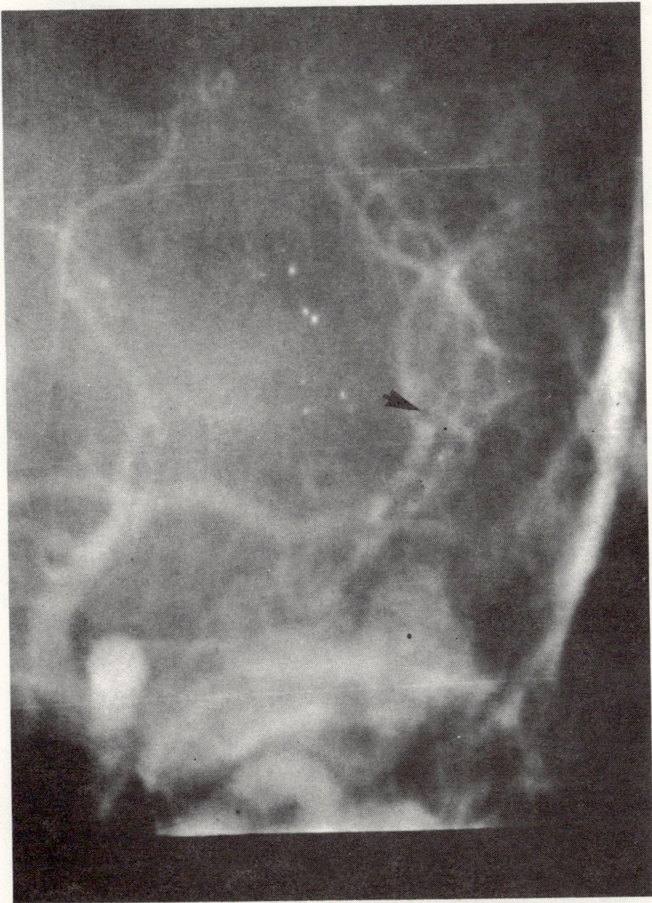

Figure 4. Left carotid angiogram in antero-posterior projection showing convex filling defect *(arrow)* at the branching of middle cerebral artery consistent with embolism.

first report, to our knowledge, of ulcers in the arteries of the posterior circulation. Three of these ulcers were in the right subclavian artery proximal to the origin of the vertebral artery (Fig. 5).

The other two ulcers were in the intraosseous segment of the vertebral artery (Fig. 6). This is a 7% incidence of ulcerated lesions in the vertebrobasilar system.

The 133 carotid arteries of the same 71 patients demonstrated 25 normal arteries, 36 smoothly stenosed, 22 irregularly stenosed,

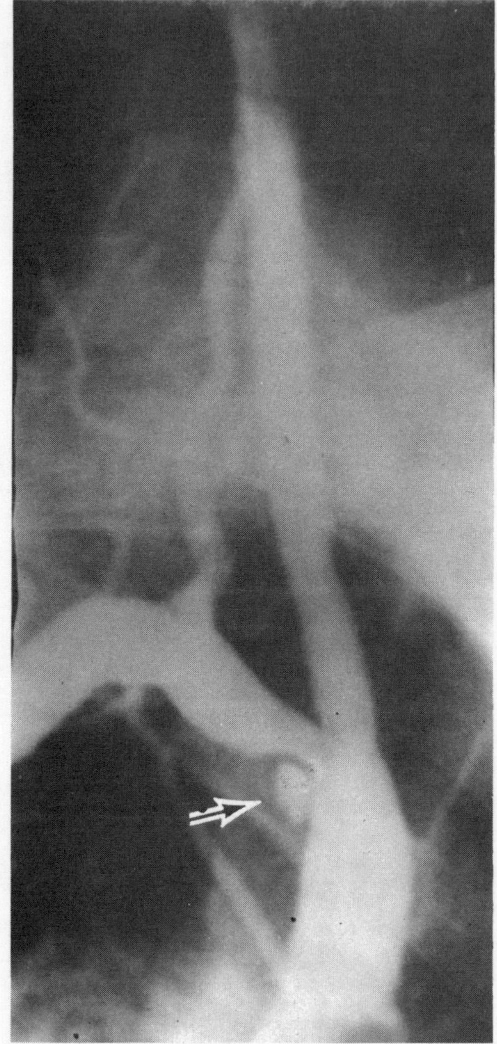

Figure 5. Right brachial angiogram revealing an ulcerated plaque in the subclavian artery just distal to the origin of common carotid artery.

and 24 ulcerated plaques (Table 1). 21 of the arteries were completely occluded and in five instances needle artifacts interfered with accurate assessment. Thus, 16% of the carotid arteries studied demonstrated ulcerated plaques.

The incidence of middle cerebral branch occlusion relative to the arteriosclerotic status of the carotid bifurcation in 82 patients

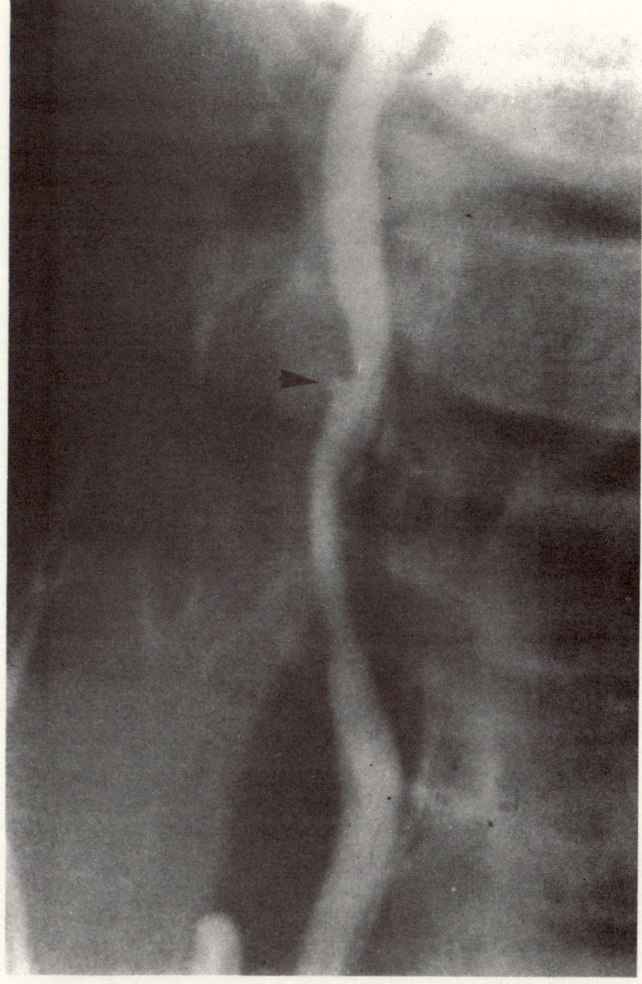

Figure 6. Left brachial angiogram on the AP-oblique view showing ulceration in the plaque of left vertebral artery *(arrow)* in the intraosseous segment.

is shown in Table 2. The 25 normal arteries and 36 smoothly stenosed arteries were placed in the same group, giving a total of 61. Middle cerebral artery occlusions were demonstrated in the territory of 10 of these carotid arteries for a 16% incidence of occlusion. Four of the branch occlusions occurred in three patients with normal carotid arteries. One of these patients had an

TABLE I

INCIDENCE OF LESIONS IN 133 EXTRACRANIAL CAROTID ARTERIES IN 71 PATIENTS.

Normal	25
Smooth Stenosis	36
Irregular Stenosis	22
Ulcerative Plaque	24
Complete Occlusions	21
Needle Artifacts	5
Total	133

TABLE II

INCIDENCE OF MIDDLE CEREBRAL BRANCH OCCLUSIONS RELATIVE TO EXTRACRANIAL VASCULAR STATUS IN 82 PATIENTS.

	No. of Carotids	MCA Occ.	% of Occ.
Normal & Smooth Stenosis	61	10	16%
Irregular Stenosis	25	11	33%
Ulcerative Plaques	36	9	

obvious cardiac source for emboli, but the other two had no evidence of either heart disease, hypertension or diabetes. Six of the occlusions occurred in five patients with smoothly stenosed carotid arteries. Two of these patients had heart disease; one had auricular fibrillation and the other had suffered a myocardial infarction ten days before the angiographic examination. A third patient in this group had a long history of diabetes and hypertension. The fourth patient with no evidence of any other systemic source of emboli showed a *cul de sac* distal to a mild carotid stenosis (Fig. 7). We felt that perhaps this *cul de sac* may well have been the site of origin of emboli.

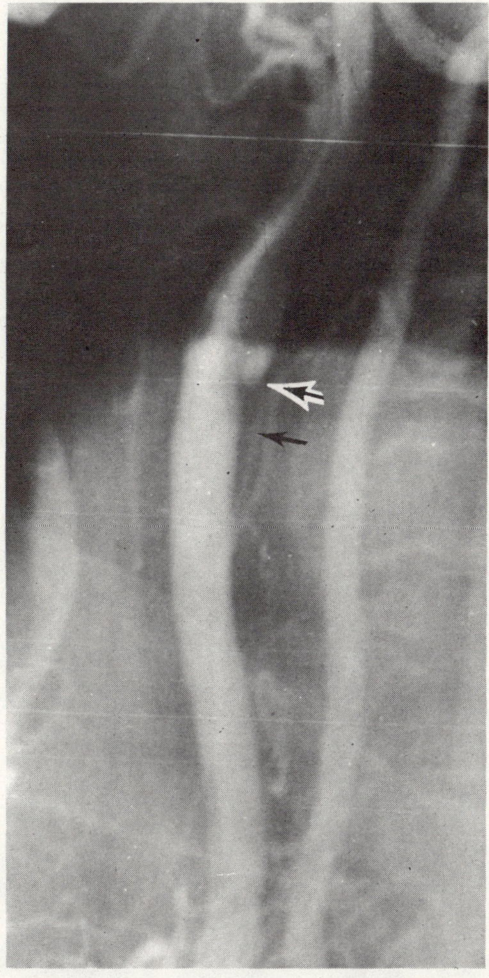

Figure 7. *'Cul de Sac' (black and white arrow)* **distal to the plaque** *(black arrow),* **best seen oblique projection of right brachial angiogram.**

Definite middle cerebral artery branch occlusions were seen in 11 of 25 angiograms with irregular stenosis, and in 9 of 36 with ulcers.

Four of the irregular plaques had a thrombus demonstrated at the bifurcation. Three of these four cases with thrombi demonstrated in their internal carotid arteries were associated with middle cerebral branch occlusions (Figs. 8A & 8B).

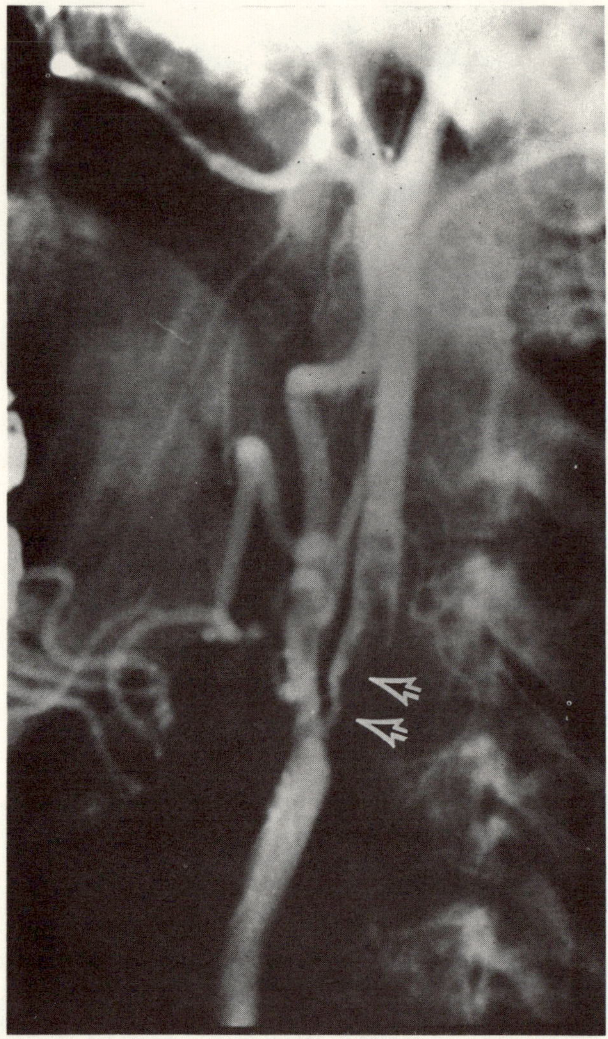

Figure 8A. A large thrombus *(arrows)* at the origin of left internal carotid artery.

Angiographic evidence of ulceration in an atheroma is not always conclusive, and the same can be said of the irregular plaque. In 11 of our 34 surgical specimens, the angiographic diagnosis was somewhat inconsistent with the surgical findings. Either an irregular plaque was seen on the angiogram, while an ulcer crater was demonstrated at surgery, or ulceration was

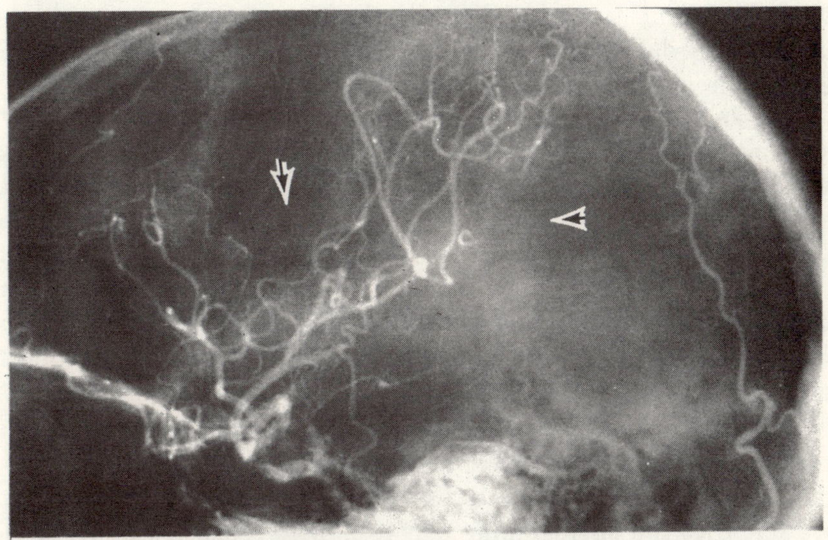

Figure 8B. Same angiogram as "A" in later phase showing multiple middle cerebral branch occlusions *(arrows)* on the lateral view.

diagnosed only to be described as an irregular plaque at exploration. The high incidence of middle cerebral artery branch occlusions associated with both irregularity and ulceration, as well as our inability to correctly separate them, has led us to evaluate these two groups together for evidence of middle cerebral branch occlusions. Of 61 ulcerated or irregular carotid plaques, 20 were associated with middle cerebral artery branch occlusions, an incidence of 33%.

Cerebral embolism secondary to a lesion in the extracranial carotid arteries is believed to be the cause of transient ischemic episodes in a majority of patients, and may frequently be the cause of more lasting neurologic deficit (1,2,5,6,7,8). If, as we believe we have demonstrated statistically, ulceration and irregularity of a carotid plaque indicate a high predisposition toward embolization, then the angiographic evaluation of the characteristics of the carotid plaque becomes as important, if not more important than the evaluation of the degree of stenosis. It may no longer be argued that it is adequate merely to faintly fill the carotid arteries and assess their degree of stenosis on a single view. Excellent contrast filling, detailed x-ray technique, multiple views and serial filming, as well as the total assessment of the intracranial circulation, is an absolute necessity.

The angiographic diagnosis of cerebral embolism depends on the size and composition of the emboli and the time lapsed since the ischemic episode. It is well known that the likelihood of detecting an embolic occlusion is very high if angiography is performed immediately following an embolic episode. In our study, most of the angiograms were performed within one to twenty days after the last episode and, therefore, the incidence of occluded vessels demonstrated is only valid on a basis relative to the condition of the carotid artery, and should not be taken as an absolute incidence. Furthermore, the diagnosis of embolic occlusion was made only when there was no evidence of local arteriosclerotic disease. While embolic occlusion may occur in these latter cases, we felt that the angiographic diagnosis here is usually conjectural. This was the case in 12 of our patients, 9 of whom had hypertension or diabetes or both. In this group, we could only definitely diagnose embolic occlusion in three. While evaluating intracranial circulation for embolic occlusion, we noted an increased incidence of narrowed or attenuated middle cerebral branches in patients who had irregular or ulcerative plaques. So, perhaps with further work we may have another sign indicating embolization.

In conclusion then, 24 ulcerated and 22 irregular plaques of the carotid arteries were demonstrated in 71 patients on 133 angiograms. It is our belief that the surgical and angiographic findings in this study suggest that the embolic implications of these lesions, that is, the irregular and the ulcerated plaques are identical. The incidence of middle cerebral branch occlusions associated with either irregular or ulcerated extracranial carotid arteries in this series is 33% as compared to 16% in cases with normal or smoothly stenosed extracranial arteries. This is a statistically significant difference at the 2% level based on Chi-square analysis.

BIBLIOGRAPHY

1. Julian, O.C., Dye, W.S., Javid, H., and Hunter, J.A.: Ulcerative lesions of the carotid artery bifurcation. *Arch. Surg.*, *86*:131-137, 1963.
2. Moore, W.S., and Hall, A.D.: Ulcerated atheroma of the carotid artery. A cause of transient cerebral ischemia. *Am. J. Surg.*, *116*:237-242, 1968.
3. Chase, N.E., and Kricheff, I.I.: Cerebral angiography in the evaluation of

patients with cerebrovascular disease. *Radiol. Clin. North America*, *4*:131-144, 1966.

4. Ring, B.A.: Diagnosis of embolic occlusions of smaller branches of the intracerebral arteries. *Am. J. Roentgenol.*, *97*: 575-582, 1966.
5. Ehrenfeld, W.F., Hoyt, W.F., and Wylie, E.J.: Embolization and transient blindness from carotid atheroma. *Arch. Surg.*, *93*:787-794, 1966.
6. Gunning, A.J., Pickering, G.W., Robb-Smith, A.H.T., and Russell, R.R.: Mural thrombosis of the internal carotid artery and subsequent embolism. *Quart. J. Med.*, *33*:155-194, 1964.
7. Hass, W.K.: "Future trends in stroke research" (Chapter IX). *In Stroke Rehabilitation*, edited by W.S. Fields and W.A. Spencer. St. Louis, Warren H. Green, Inc., 119-137, 1967.
8. Millikan, C.H.: The pathogenesis of transient focal cerebral ischemia. *Circulation*, *32*:438-450, 1965.

Chapter IV

ULCERATED ATHEROSCLEROTIC LESIONS IN THE CAROTID BIFURCATION*

WILLIAM K. EHRENFELD, M.D.

We have long been interested in ulcerated atherosclerotic lesions at the carotid bifurcation, although published reports from other centers, as well as our own, have somewhat belatedly called attention to the relationship of ulcerated lesions to cerebrovascular insufficiency states (1-4). My remarks will concern the pathogenesis of these ulcerated atheromas, their relation to transient cerebral ischemia and stroke, and how these factors influence the vascular surgeon.

Ulceration of atherosclerotic lesions at the carotid bifurcation is common in comparison to ulceration at other sites. Although atherosclerosis is a diffuse disease, it usually becomes clinically manifest in focal areas of arterial stenosis involving, among others, the coronary arteries, renal and visceral arteries, terminal aorta and superficial femoral arteries. However, for reasons that are not clear, ulceration of these vessels in comparison to the extracranial arteries is uncommon.

The pathogenesis of atherosclerotic ulceration is quite different from the previously mentioned ulceration of the gastro-intestinal tract. Duodenal ulcer disease begins with ulceration of the mucosa, with extension into the sub-mucosa or serosa. We believe that in most instances atherosclerotic ulceration begins with a subintimal hemorrhage which encroaches upon the arterial lumen, which may then cause intimal necrosis and ulceration. Cerebral or ocular embolization may result from discharge of atherosclerotic debris

*From the Vascular Surgery Service, University of California Medical Center, San Francisco, California.

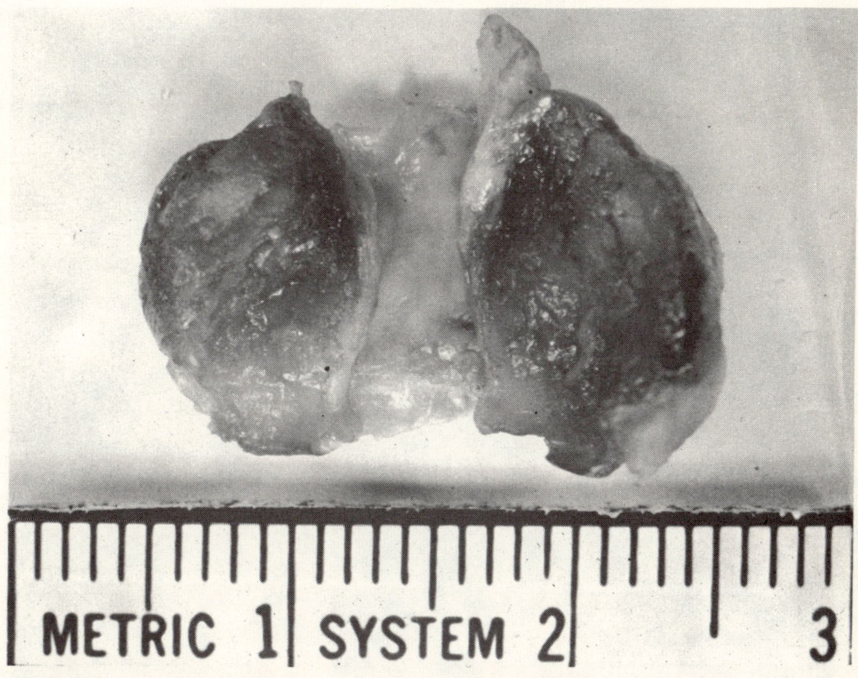

Figure 1. Surgical specimen showing narrowing of the arterial lumen and expansion of the bulb from a recent subintimal hemorrhage. The intimal surface is intact. (From Wylie, E.J., and Ehrenfeld, W.K., *Extracranial Occlusive Cerebrovascular Disease,* Philadelphia, W.B. Saunders Co., 1970, p. 40.)

into the bloodstream itself. Thrombosis or further embolization may follow the appearance of formed blood elements, including platelet aggregates, on the ulcerated surface.

The pathogenesis and manifestations of arterial ulceration at the carotid bifurcation are illustrated by the following case reports and accompanying photographs.

Case 1. A 57-year-old farmer was admitted with a history of abrupt onset of postural lightheadedness. Aortic arch arteriography showed occlusion of the left internal carotid artery and stenosis of the right internal carotid artery. A right carotid endarterectomy was performed (Fig. 1).

Case 2. A 63-year-old housewife had several episodes of transient blindness in the right eye and two episodes of

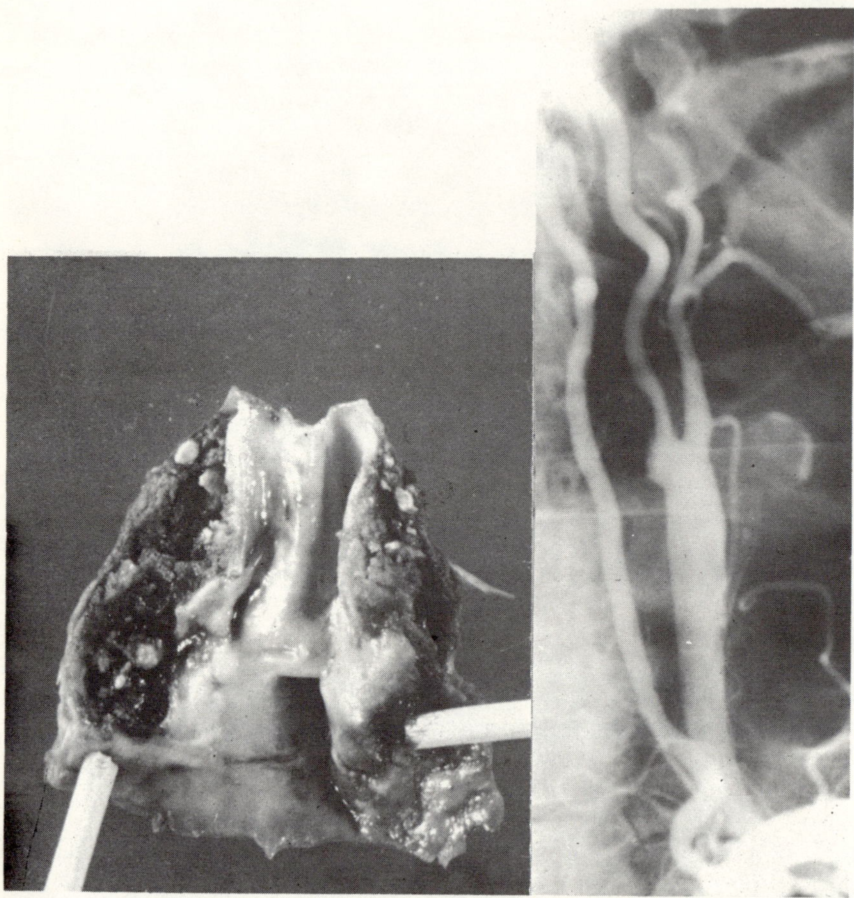

Figure 2. *Left:* **Specimen removed by endarterectomy showing intramural hemorrhage and intimal ulceration.** *Right:* Carotid and vertebral arteriogram showing a shallow ulcerated area in the distal portion of the common carotid artery in the absence of significant luminal narrowing. (*Ibid.*, p. 32).

dyssynchronous transient left hemiparesis. A right carotid endarterectomy was performed (Fig. 2). The transient ischemic attacks ceased after operation. In all likelihood the attacks were caused by embolization to the ipsilateral retina and hemisphere. The emboli were probably composed of atherosclerotic debris and blood elements discharged from the ulcer crater.

Case 3. A 71-year-old lady had a carotid endarterectomy for numerous TIA's. A typical ulcerated carotid atheroma was found

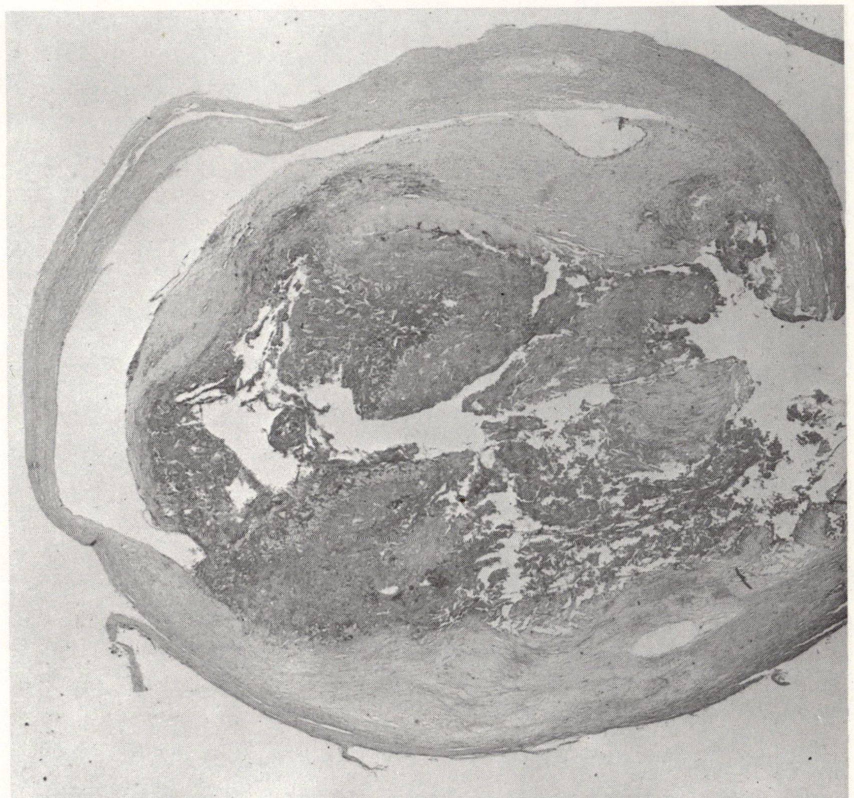

Figure 3. Low power photomicrograph of an ulcerated carotid atheroma in which there is a circumferential ulcer filled with atherosclerotic debris, including organizing thrombus and multiple cholesterol clefts. (From Ehrenfeld, W.K., Hoyt, W.F., and Wylie, E.J., *Arch. Surg., 93*:787, 1966.)

at operation (Fig. 3). A retinal photograph of this patient showed two distinct emboli (Fig. 4). Presumably, these emboli originated at the ipsilateral carotid bifurcation.

Case 4. A right carotid arteriogram was performed in a 52-year-old man who had developed a prolonged left hemiparesis after numerous transient hemiparetic attacks. After the patient's condition stabilized and he recovered, an ulcerated carotid atheroma was removed by endarterectomy.

With continued experience and observation, vascular surgeons are recognizing the importance of cerebral and ocular embolization. We have learned that in patients who have focal transient

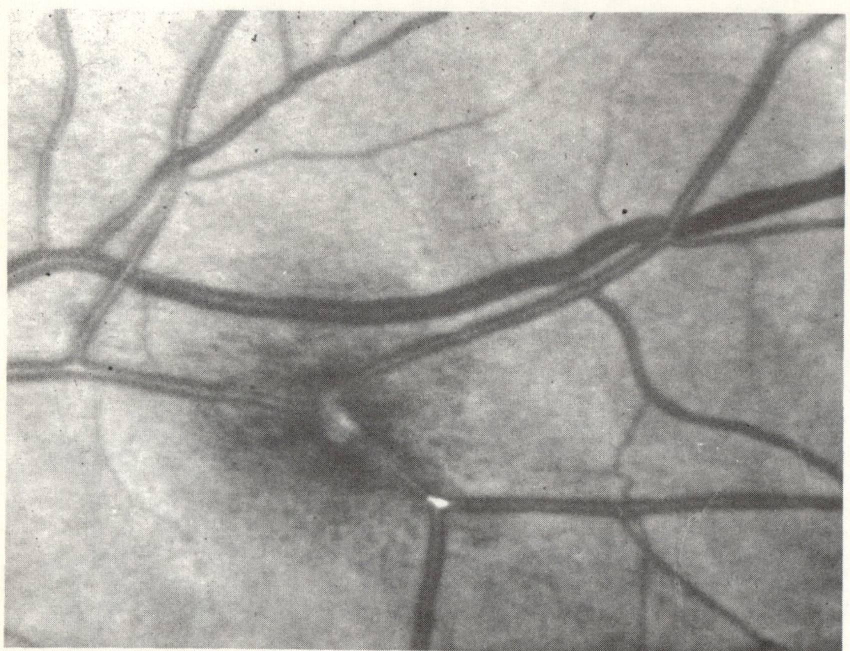

Figure 4. Cholesterol retinal emboli in the right eye of Case 3. These emboli are lodged at arteriolar bifurcations. The proximal embolus has caused a retinal hemorrhage. *(Ibid.)*

attacks, significant luminal stenosis is not a necessary pre-requisite to surgical intervention. When ulceration and embolization are suspected, then the degree of luminal narrowing is unimportant. The eyegrounds in all patients with TIA's are examined for telltale emboli. It is recognized, however, that retinal emboli are visible at the time of examination in only a small number of patients since most have been washed into the venous system. We have also stopped using the test of carotid compression for fear of dislodging thrombo-embolic material.

Vascular surgeons have come to recognize that the potentially ulcerated carotid atheroma must be handled very carefully at operation. Early in our experience, when we performed carotid endarterectomy under local anesthesia, several patients abruptly developed neurological deficits prior to occlusion by arterial clamping. When the lesion was later examined at operation, irregular intimal ulceration was seen. It is probable that emboli

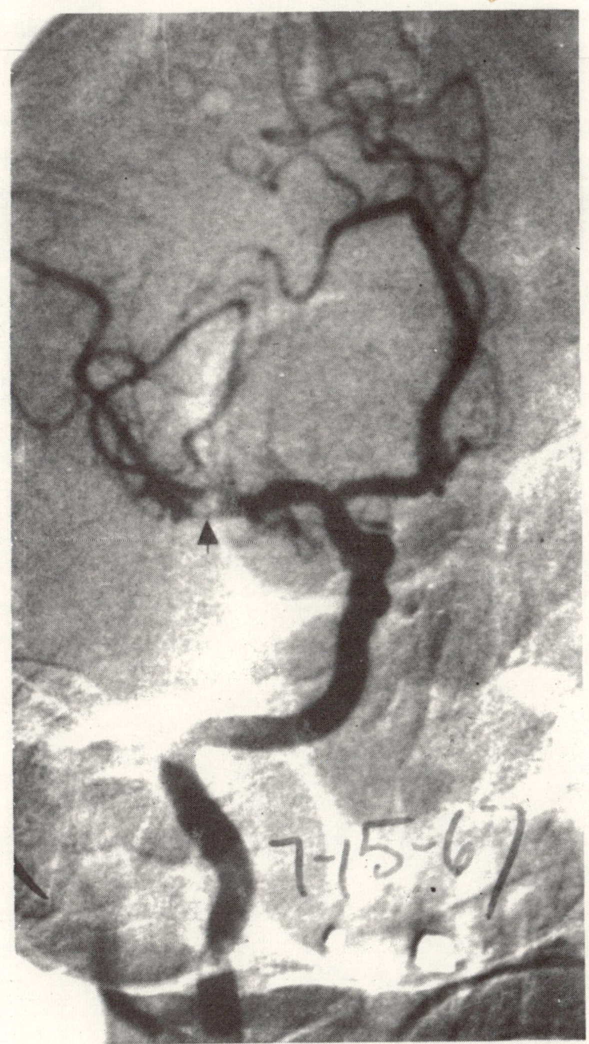

Figure 5. Right carotid arteriogram showing a macroembolus in the right middle cerebral artery (*arrow*). (Wylie and Ehrenfeld, Op. cit., p. 39).

dislodged during the initial dissection caused the neurological deficits.

In summary, I agree with the previous speakers that thrombo-embolic phenomena are very important in certain cerebrovascular insufficiency states. I do not believe, however, that all transient ischemic attacks are caused by this mechanism. It is important to recognize that patients with focal transient ischemic attacks respond very well to carotid revascularization surgery, both in terms of relief of existing disability caused by transient attacks and prophylaxis to prevent stroke.

REFERENCES

1. Julian, O.C., Dye, W.S., Javid, H., and Hunter, J.A.: Ulcerative lesions of the carotid artery bifurcation. *Arch. Surg., 86*:803-809, 1963.
2. Gunning, A.J., Pickering, G.W., Robb-Smith, A.H.T., and Russell, R.W.R.: Mural thrombosis of the internal carotid artery and subsequent embolism. *Quart. J. Med., 33*:155-195, 1964.
3. Ehrenfeld, W.K., Hoyt, W.F., and Wylie, E.J.: Embolization and transient blindness from carotid atheroma. *Arch. Surg., 93*:787-794, 1966.
4. Wylie, E.J., and Ehrenfeld, W.K.: *Extracranial Occlusive Cerebrovascular Disease, Diagnosis and Management.* W.B. Saunders 1970.

Chapter V

EMBOLI FROM THE CAROTID BIFURCATION IN THE PATHOGENESIS OF CEREBRAL ISCHEMIC ATTACKS

WESLEY S. MOORE, M.D.

Since the original description of carotid artery reconstruction by Eastcott, Pickering and Rob (1), many hundreds of patients have been relieved of neurological symptoms by carotid endarterectomy. The causal relationship between extracranial arteriosclerosis and transient neurological dysfunction has been well established; however, the exact mechanism by which extracranial atheroma induce neurological sequelae remains controversial. The two major explanations for this phenomenon are the arterial stenotic and the arterial embolic theories.

The arterial stenotic theory would explain neurological symptoms on the basis of reduced cerebral blood flow through a critical stenosis. A critical stenosis is defined as that degree of stenosis which produces a pressure gradient across the lesion. The embolic theory envisions the carotid bifurcation atheroma as a potential source for thrombotic, atheromatous, or platelet aggregate material which, because of its strategic location, can fragment and embolize the brain.

Many vascular surgeons have accepted the arterial stenotic theory as an explanation for transient cerebral dysfunction. This is perhaps due to the readily apparent analogy to peripheral vascular insufficiency. However, on closer examination there are a number of events peculiar to transient cerebral ischemic attacks which cannot be explained by the stenotic theory alone.

1) If the symptoms of transient cerebral dysfunction are due to a period of reduced cerebral blood flow through a stenotic vessel, why is it that 90% of patients with neurological symptoms secondary to extracranial vascular disease easily tolerate total

occlusion of the carotid artery as observed under local anesthesia during its repair? (2).

2) A 50% reduction in cross sectional area of the carotid artery is capable of producing a pressure gradient; however, clinical and laboratory studies have demonstrated that a stenosis of at least 90% is necessary to reduce blood flow through the internal carotid artery (3,4). Why is it that many patients with lesions significantly less than 90% have their symptoms of transient cerebral dysfunction dramatically relieved by removal of these "subcritical" stenoses?

3) When a high-grade stenosis of the internal carotid artery progresses to total occlusion, the patient may have a stroke or the event may occur without any symptoms whatsoever. Why is it that patients with transient ischemic attacks, who sustain asymptomatic occlusion of the carotid artery, will have a concomitant cessation of their attacks of transient cerebral dysfunction? (5,6).

4) The transient nature of cerebral dysfunction in association with a constant demand for cerebral blood flow in the presence of a rigid stenosis has been explained as occurring with intermittent drops of systemic arterial blood pressure (7,8). Why is it that transient ischemic attacks are not reproduced with the deliberate lowering of systemic blood pressure by hypotensive agents? (1.9).

5) If a carotid artery stenosis reduces cerebral blood flow, why then can one not document increase in cerebral blood flow following its repair (11), or experimentally measure a reduction in hemispheric blood flow when a critical stenosis is introduced? (4).

6) Since chronic anticoagulant therapy has no effect on the rheologic properties of blood, why then is there a significant decrease in the incidence of transient cerebral dysfunction among patients who are treated with chronic anticoagulation therapy in comparison to a control group? (12).

Because of these unanswered questions, it has been necessary to explore other possible explanations of transient cerebral dysfunction associated with extracranial vascular disease. While embolization to the brain from mural thrombus on a carotid bifurcation atheroma was demonstrated as early as 1905 by Chiari (13), it was only recently that attention has been refocused on this mechanism as an explanation for transient cerebral ischemia. In 1963, Julian and his associates reviewed a series of carotid operations in which 17 cases were identified with ulcerative atheromatous stenoses at the time of operation. In their opinion, these lesions were capable of releasing emboli to the brain (14). In the same year, the British neurologist Gunning and his co-workers reviewed the subject of transient cerebral dysfunction and presented several additional cases with mural thrombosis and documented embolization to the brain. These authors proposed that the embolic theory was the best explanation for transient cerebral dysfunction associated with extracranial vascular disease (15).

Additional evidence in support of the embolic theory comes from visualization of embolic material in the retinal vessels of patients with amaurosis fugax and ipsilateral carotid artery lesions (16-18). The fact that the number of transient ischemic attacks can be reduced by anticoagulant therapy suggests that there must be some mechanism associated with the thrombotic process that is operational in the production of transient dysfunction. The observation that asymptomatic total occlusion of the internal carotid artery will stop transient ischemic attacks suggests that the mechanism of transient ischemia is embolic, and that occlusion of the vessel simply obstructs the pathway of embolic particles from the carotid bifurcation atheroma to the brain. In spite of the evidence in favor of the embolic theory, it has been difficult to prove on the basis of the current operative experience because of the generally accepted criteria of arterial stenosis for operative selection. Many surgeons have argued, therefore, that the good postoperative results following carotid endarterectomy are explained by augmented blood flow when stenotic lesions are removed.

Several years ago it occurred to us that if the embolic theory was correct, then the percentage of stenosis in an extracranial vessel should not be the major consideration in selecting patients for operation. According to this theory, any roughened or ulcerated atheromatous lesion, regardless of size, could be an embolic source. If one elected, therefore, not to operate on patients with transient ischemic attacks simply because a high-grade stenosis was not present, one might be overlooking a source of emboli and the opportunity to effectively prevent further ischemic attacks. In 1967, we presented our experience with nine patients undergoing carotid endarterectomy for non-stenotic, ulcerated lesions of the carotid bifurcation with total relief of hemispheric symptoms (19). It was our contention that the data provided additional evidence in support of the embolic theory, since removal of these non-stenotic lesions could not be construed as having increased blood flow. At the present time, we have expanded our series and have had the opportunity to increase the duration of post-operative follow-up.

From September 1966 through December 1969, 35 patients underwent 49 carotid endarterectomies. The majority of the patients are in the seventh and eight decades, with ages ranging from 44 to 76 years. Of the 35 patients in this series, 31 presented with episodes of transient neurological dysfunction, ten had concomitant history of completed stroke, and four had completed stroke as their only manifestation of cerebrovascular disease. The distribution of transient ischemic attacks is as follows: 15 patients had motor ischemic attacks, 4 patients had sensory ischemic attacks, 7 patients had episodes of amaurosis fugax, and 10 patients had nonlateralizing symptoms such as dizziness, vertigo, syncope, or nonspecific blurring of vision. Six of 10 patients had these symptoms as their only manifestation of cerebral dysfunction, while 4 patients had these symptoms in association with lateralizing findings.

On physical examination only 13 patients, or 37%, had a carotid bruit; 11 patients had a modest residual paresis, and 2 patients had partial visual field loss.

Aortocranial angiography revealed unilateral carotid ulceration in 23 patients and bilateral carotid ulceration in 12 patients; 6 patients had associated stenoses or occlusions of other extracranial vessels in addition to their ulcerative nonstenotic lesions.

Fourteen patients underwent bilateral carotid endarterectomy and 21 patients underwent unilateral carotid endarterectomy, for a total of 49 operations in 35 patients.

Thirty-one patients underwent 45 operations without death or complications. Of the remaining 4 patients, one died as a result of his operation. This was due to injudicious use of hypotensive agents in the treatment of a postoperative hypertensive episode. Three patients had episodes of transient monoparesis at the time the carotid artery was mobilized, presumably from embolization which occurred as a result of manipulation of the carotid bifurcation. None of these three patients experienced permanent deficit. There were no completed strokes as a complication of this operation.

Follow-up has ranged from 4 to 39 months, with a mean follow-up of 23 months. Of the initial 35 patients having operations, 29 are currently living at the time of this report. There was one postoperative death and five late deaths: four from myocardial infarction and one from carcinoma of the lung. Follow-up evaluation is current in all living patients. Of the five late deaths, all were followed at frequent intervals prior to death.

In analyzing the results of operation on the relief of specific symptoms of the 13 patients experiencing motor transient ischemic attacks, 11 were asymptomatic, one developed a late false aneurysm, and one had a late stroke on the opposite side. A retrospective review of this patient's arteriograms revealed an ulcerative lesion of the opposite carotid artery. It was elected not to operate on that second side because the patient was asymptomatic at the time of his initial evaluation. Four patients with sensory ischemic attacks are all asymptomatic. Of seven patients with amaurosis, all are asymptomatic; and of ten patients with nonlateralizing symptoms, seven have been relieved of their symptoms and three continue to have nonlateralizing symptoms. Thus, 35 patients underwent 49 carotid endarterectomies. The relief of hemispheric transient ischemic attacks during the follow-up period was 100%; the relief of nonlateralizing symptoms, however, was only 70%.

In summary then, we have reviewed the two major theories of transient cerebral ischemia, that is, the arterial stenotic and arterial embolic theories. The evidence presented suggests that total relief of hemispheric attacks follows removal of nonstenotic, ulcerated lesions, and adds further support to the embolic theory.

REFERENCES

1. Eastcott, H.H.G., Pickering, G.W., and Rob, C.G.: Reconstruction of internal carotid artery in a patient with intermittent attacks of hemiplegia. *Lancet, 2*:994-996, 1954.
2. Moore, W.S., and Hall, A.D.: Carotid artery back pressure. A test of cerebral tolerance to temporary carotid occlusion. *Arch. Surg., 99*:702-710, 1969.

3. Brice, J.G., Dowsett, D.J., and Lowe, R.D.: Haemodynamic effects of carotid artery stenosis. *Brit. Med. J.*, *2*:1363-1366, 1964.

4. Eklof, B., and Schwartz, S.I.: Effects of critical stenosis of the carotid artery and compromised cephalic blood flow. *Arch. Surg.*, *99*:695-701, 1969.

5. Russell, R.W., and Cranston, W.I.: Ophthalmodynamometry in carotid artery disease. *J. Neurol. Neurosurg. Psychiat.*, *24*:281-286, 1961.

6. Drake, W.E. Jr., and Drake, M.A.L.: Clinical and angiographic correlates of cerebrovascular insufficiency. *Amer. J. Med.*, *45*:253-270, 1968.

7. Denny-Brown, D.: Recurrent cerebrovascular episodes. *Arch. Neurol.*, *2*:194-210, 1960.

8. Corday, E., Rothenberg, S., and Weiner, S.M.: Cerebral vascular insufficiency: an explanation of the transient stroke. *Arch. Int. Med.*, *98*:683-690, 1956.

9. Kendall R.E., and Marshall, J.: Role of hypotension in the genesis of transient focal cerebral ischaemic attacks. *Brit. Med. J.*, *2*:344-348, 1963.

10. Fazekas, J.F., and Alman, R.W.: The role of hypotension in transitory focal cerebral ischemia. *Amer. J. Med. Sci.*, *248*:567-570, 1964.

11. Adams, J.E., Smith, M.C., and Wylie, E.J.: Cerebral blood flow and hemodynamics in extracranial vascular disease: effect of endarterectomy. *Surgery*, *53*:449-455, 1963.

12. Fisher, C.M.: Anticoagulant therapy in cerebral thrombosis and cerebral embolism. *Neurology (Minneap)*, *11*:119-131, 1961.

13. Chiari, H.: Ueber das Verhalten des Teilungswinkels der Carotis communis bei der Endarteriitis chronica deformans. *Verh. Deutsch. Ges. Path.*, *9*:326-330, 1905.

14. Julian, O.C., Dye, W.S., Javid, H. et al: Ulcerative lesions of the carotid artery bifurcation. *Arch. Surg.*, *86*:803-809, 1963.

15. Gunning, A.J., Pickering, G.W., Robb-Smith, A.H.T. et al: Mural thrombosis of the internal carotid artery and subsequent embolism. *Quart. J. Med.*, *33*:155-195, 1964.

16. Fisher, C.M.: Observations of the fundus oculi in transient monocular blindness. *Neurology (Minneap)*, 9:333-347,1959.

17. Hollenhorst, R.W.: Significance of bright plaques in the retinal arterioles. *JAMA*, *178*:23-29, 1961.

18. Ehrenfeld, W.K., Hoyt, W.F., and Wylie, E.J.: Embolization and transient blindness from carotid atheroma. Surgical considerations. *Arch. Surg.*, *93*:787-794, 1966.

19. Moore, W.S., and Hall, A.D.: Ulcerated atheroma of the carotid artery. A major cause of transient cerebral ischemia. *Amer. J. Surg.*, *116*:237-242, 1968.

DISCUSSION OF CHAPTERS I THROUGH V

Dr. William S. Fields, Houston, Tex.: Our essayists to this point have provided us with background information regarding transient cerebral ischemic attacks and their relationship to lesions in the cervical extracranial arteries. It should be evident that there is still some disagreement with regard to the pathogenesis of these phenomena, as well as some uncertainty regarding appropriate therapeutic measures which should be taken for their relief.

Among the neurologists, neurosurgeons and vascular surgeons who have had sufficient experience with arterial reconstructive operations, there is a reasonable concensus of opinion. These operations have been successful in the clinical management of patients with carotid lesions producing a stenosis of greater than 50%. However, there is still considerable uncertainty regarding operation in patients in whom the lesions are non-obstructing but may, nevertheless, be the source of thromboembolism.

Dr. Clark Millikan has had a long-time interest in this aspect of cerebrovascular disease. He was among the first to describe these attacks in explicit detail and to recognize the importance of intra-arterial thromboembolism. I would appreciate his opening the discussion of these papers.

Dr. Clark Millikan, Rochester, Minn.: Since this conference particularly concerns aspirin or any kind of platelet aggregation inhibiting agents, a succinct way to summarize ideas about the pathogenesis of transient focal cerebral ischemic attacks is to quote from an article of November 30, 1955, which I wrote with Doctors Siekert and Shick:[1] "Our present concept of the pathogenesis of attacks is as follows: A thrombus begins to form on an area of diseased endothelium. This soft material may reach a size

[1]Millikan, C.H., Siekert, R.G., and Shick, R.M.: Studies in cerebrovascular disease. V. The use of anticoagulant drugs in the treatment of intermittent insufficiency of the internal carotid arterial system. *Proc. Staff Meet. of Mayo Clinic, 30*:578-586 (Nov. 30) 1955.

sufficient to produce enough alteration in blood flow to cause symptoms, break from its source, fragment and be carried away. More likely, however, appears the possibility that the newly formed clot becomes dislodged before symptoms occur, travels to a place where the vessels branch, lodges for a few minutes (symptoms produced) and then fragments and is carried away."

In presenting the Lewis A. Conner Memorial Lecture at the annual meeting of the American Heart Association in 1961, I summarized the various items which may enter into the pathogenesis of transient focal cerebral ischemia.[2] These items included: vasospasm, transitory systemic hypotension, kinking or compression of an artery, polycythemia, severe anemia, transitory hypoglycemia, transitory shunts and, finally, the major category of thrombosis or emboli secondary to or associated with atherosclerosis. Thus, it has been repeatedly emphasized that the character of the atherosclerosis developing in the basilar artery with marked roughening of the intima and occasional ulceration appears along with laminations of clot found in patients coming to autopsy with basilar thrombosis and cerebral infarction. It then becomes logical to speculate that beginning thrombosis, at the orifice of a circumferential basilar branch, might well change flow patterns for a few minutes, only to have normal flow restored when the lytic process effectively destroyed the beginning clot. It has even been speculated that minute atherosclerotic lesions in the initial portions of the penetrating branches of the middle cerebral artery, or close to the orifice of circumferential branches of the basilar artery, might be the site of transient clot formation and thus constitute an additional mechanism for the production of transient ischemic attacks. Recently, Dr. Miller Fisher displayed such a lesion.[3] By a diligent search of thousands of sections, taking countless hours, he found significant atherosclerotic lesions at the beginning portion of penetrating branches of the middle cerebral artery. In one slide, there was a fresh thrombus forming on the distal portion of such an atherosclerotic lesion.

---

[2]Millikan, C.H.: The Pathogenesis of transient focal cerebral ischemia. The Lewis A. Conner Memorial Lecture, presented at the 34th Scientific Sessions of the American Heart Association, Miami, Fla., Oct. 1961. *Circulation, 32*:438-450, 1965.

[3]Fisher, C. Miller: Basilar artery branch infarction. *Neurology*, in press, 1970.

Thus, we have heard summarized today observations which have been made for as long as 15 years--observations which point to the potential importance of changing the clotting mechanism in order to prevent transient ischemic attacks. The importance and, perhaps, the unique contribution of changing this clotting mechanism may come by way of decreasing the adhesiveness of platelets. Therefore, it seems highly appropriate for us to discuss the possible advantages of a drug such as aspirin.

Dr. Fields: It becomes increasingly obvious that we can no longer seriously accept a unitary theory of the pathogenesis of transient cerebral ischemic attacks. Dr. Moore's argument in favor of one mechanism, which he described so beautifully, certainly has points in its favor. However, I would question his statement that other mechanisms than thromboembolism might be excluded on the basis of certain physiologic phenomena. I am not quite prepared to accept this proposition.

Dr. William K. Hass, New York, N. Y.: A question should be raised about the validity of Dr. Ehrenfeld's postulate that bleeding into the plaque is a necessary prerequisite for ulceration. I am not certain, from our own experience, that subintimal bleeding, or bleeding into the plaque, is the only mechanism for plaque ulceration. I know of no serial studies on this point, nor are they really possible, save through a retrospective gathering of data from many sources.

We have found, for instance, at surgery, in a patient who had had emboli to the ipsilateral retina, a carotid plaque which had only a pinhole-size opening. There was no evidence of bleeding, and tiny amounts of friable cholesterol material were coming out of the opening.

Since we have Dr. Moore here, as well as Dr. Ehrenfeld, I wonder if Dr. Moore has his own concept of what leads to ulceration, and whether it varies from Dr. Ehrenfeld's?

Dr. Wesley S. Moore, San Francisco, Calif.: I am sure that bleeding into an arteriosclerotic plaque is certainly an important mechanism in the degeneration of an atheromatous lesion; however, it is certainly not the only mechanism. Many of the atheromatous lesions that we have looked at do, for some reason or another, undergo degeneration. While an arteriosclerotic plaque does not have a blood supply, it is similar to a tumor which enlarges and undergoes central necrosis because of lack of nutrition. In the case of a plaque, it becomes softened, the surface endothelium sloughs, and the contents of the softened plaque break out and embolize downstream. This mechanism not only explains ulceration, but may also explain a major neurologic manifestation in association with the process of embolization.

Dr. Hass: In other words, it is really a matter of chance whether the grumous material causes a transient cerebral ischemic attack or frank cerebral infarction, or whether, when the ulceration develops, attempted repair with platelet aggregation is the cause. This leads us into the difficulty of trying to analyze drug effects in the presence of a complex pathogenetic mechanism.

Dr. Edward B. Truitt, Columbus, O.: Since we seem to be in the process of putting on the agenda some possible causes of transitory ischemic attacks, I would like to introduce some biochemical ideas which occur to pharmacologists. I should hate to wait until later, only to find that they have not been presented.

My own pharmacologic viewpoint is characterized by a segment of pharmacology known as "catecholamania pharmacologica." I am, therefore, inclined toward ideas about what happens following the breakdown of platelets and other events occuring in clotting to suggest certain biogenic amine influences which would involve the release of vasospastic or vasoactive compounds. Serotonin, or 5-hydroxytryptamine, particularly, has to be considered as one of the substances that could be released and delivered at the site of this lesion, as well as downstream, with probable vascular effects.

I am reminded that pharmacologists probably have been, in the laboratory at least, some of the most active manipulators of the carotid artery, especially in dogs. We have ligated them, cannulated them, clamped them, and everything else. Thus, we are very familiar with the neurogenic vasomotor effects following any sort of trauma to the artery, with the production of temporary ischemia under a variety of circumstances.

Also, I would like to have considered the possibility of the release of biogenic amines, as well as other polypeptides and vasoactive substances which could evolve in the coagulation process.

Dr. Hass: We are fortunate to have with us Dr. Marjorie Zucker and Dr. Aaron Marcus, who have written an excellent volume on platelet physiology.[4] I wonder if either of them would care to comment on what might be released by platelet lysozymes, or other organelles, which might cause necrosis and ulceration.

Dr. Marjorie B. Zucker, New York, N. Y.: It is an enticing idea to think that serotonin released from platelets might cause vasoconstriction. However, I am not convinced that it occurs, for two reasons: First of all, human platelets contain quite a low amount of serotonin, compared with many animal species; and secondly, as far as I know, nobody has been able to show that a platelet thrombus inside a vessel can cause vasoconstriction. Perhaps the serotonin does not get through the wall of the vessel to the smooth muscle very well. If the serotonin is released outside the vessel, I showed a long time ago that you can get very impressive vasoconstriction, at least in animals.[5] I am not convinced that if you have a platelet thrombus inside a vessel, you can get vasoconstriction around it, and I would be curious to know if anybody has evidence to the contrary.

Dr. William K. Ehrenfeld, San Francisco, Calif.: In answer to the question that was originally raised, I would not want to say that subintimal hemorrhage is the only cause for eventual intimal ulceration of the carotid bifurcation. I think it is probably the most important and most common cause of ulceration at the carotid bifurcation, but I would agree with Dr. Moore that one may have intimal ulceration alone, probably as a result of ischemia within the intima itself. Surface deposition of blood elements would then follow.

I also agree with Dr. Fields that ulceration and embolization are not the only cause for cerebral ischemia. I base this upon our study of carotid lesions in over 70 patients who had transient retinal blindness, or amaurosis fugax, as their presenting pre-operative complaint. In these patients, who had "pure" symptoms of carotid insufficiency, it was possible to predict one

---

[4]Marcus. A.J., and Zucker, M.B., *The Physiology of Blood Platelets.* New York and London: Grune & Stratton, 1965.

[5]Zucker, M.B.: Platelet agglutination and vasoconstriction as factors in spontaneous hemostasis in normal, thrombocyteopenic, heparinized and hypoprothrombinemic rats. *Amer. J. Physiol.,148*:275-288, 1947.

of two types of lesions at the carotid bifurcation. They had either an ulcerated lesion accompanied by any degree of stenosis, or even no stenosis, or there was a very severe stenosis without intimal ulceration at the carotid bifurcation. I can tell you that a substantial number of these patients with very severe stenosis had no evidence of ulceration. These were smooth atheromas that were severely stenotic. I do not know whether or not embolization can occur because of slow flow or the eddy currents distal to the stenosis, followed by release of emboli, but certainly at operation one can find a substantial number of lesions that are purely smooth. Moreover, patients with attacks of transient monocular blindness are the ones who have the purest form of transient ischemic attack. I think we should recognize the possibility, or even probability, that certain forms of cerebral ischemia are not the result of ulceration and subsequent embolization.

Dr. Fields: I have one further comment which bears upon the problem of the direction in which a branch artery takes off from its parent vessel. Certainly, ophthalmic arteries of many individuals take off at a rather acute angle, and may be almost opposite to the direction of carotid flow in some, yet emboli seem to get into these vessels without too great difficulty.

Another important fact which should be mentioned at this juncture relates to the appearance of emboli in the retinal vessels immediately following carotid endarterectomy. Once a plaque is removed by this surgical procedure, there is left behind a raw surface upon which aggregates of blood elements accumulate. If one goes to the recovery room immediately following surgery and examines the fundus of the eye on the operated side, platelet or fibrinoplatelet emboli will almost invariably be observed in the retinal arteries.[6] In spite of this fact, these patients rarely complain of visual disturbance, and there are only infrequent serious sequelae, certainly few of a permanent nature.

Dr. Hass: I suspect we will hear a good deal later from Dr. Weiss about post-operative experimental thrombosis or thromboembolism. He has done an interesting study on endarterectomy

[6] Wylie, E.J.: Discussion of papers by Fields, W.S., and Bauer, R.B., *et al.*, page 264. *In* Millikan, C.H., Siekert, R.B., and Whisnant, J.P. (eds): *Cerebral Vascular Disease, Transactions of the Fifth Conference*, New York, Grune & Stratton, 1966.

and thrombosis and the effects of aspirin pre-treatment.

It would be helpful at this point to have Dr. Kricheff summarize the radiographic aspects of our problem, since arteriography must play a very significant role in any future study.

Dr. Irvin I. Kricheff, New York, N.Y.: I feel somewhat plebeian in the face of all this science. Basically, my function, as a radiologist, has been, and will continue to be, to study these individuals with a view to providing criteria for the selection of patients for further investigation. I mentioned in my talk that these patients will have to be studied by detailed angiographic techniques that clearly show segments of stenotic arteries in profile.

One thing that becomes obvious is that many of the ancillary studies that have come and gone in this field, such as ultrasound, thermography, and ophthalmodynamometry, are pretty much out of business in the "year of the ulcerated plaque." Perhaps in addition to angiography, retinal photography of some kind might be useful in any projected study.

The last problem which Dr. Fields alluded to at the outset is the classic criterion of 30% stenosis that was used in the national cooperative study. It is my recollection that we wanted to operate on all stenoses and that 30% was selected as that degree at which nobody would call a normal artery abnormal and proceed to operate. It was a safety factor for patients. I do not believe that anybody felt that 30% was a magic figure.

What do we do now when we say that any type of irregularity or ulceration is potentially dangerous? How do we draw the very fine line in order to avoid the significant clinical problem of operating on people whose arteries are not truly irregular? If you include people who don't really have irregular vessels, how are they going to fit into your study? This is something that I think will require much more detailed discussion.

Dr. Hass: We are not just going to operate; we are considering medical therapy as well.

PART II

INHIBITION OF PLATELET AGGREGATION

Moderator

Anthony P. Fletcher, M.D.

Chapter VI

THE EFFECTS OF ASPIRIN ON PLATELETS AND THROMBOSIS

An Historical Review and Experimental Studies*

HARVEY J. WEISS, M.D.

I would like to thank Doctors Fields and Hass for inviting me to speak at this first "International Symposium on Neuro-hematology." I think it is interesting to note that aspirin, which has been used extensively for treating minor headaches, is now being considered as a prophylaxis against headaches of a more serious nature.

Previous speakers at this conference have indicated that transient attacks of cerebral ischemia may be due to embolization of platelet aggregates which have formed at the site of ulcerated atherosclerotic plaques. The object of this meeting is to explore the possibility that such attacks might be reduced by an agent which inhibits the formation of a platelet aggregate. Although our knowledge concerning the mechanism of platelet aggregation is still very incomplete, several facts appear to be reasonably well established.

First, platelets do not ordinarily adhere to or aggregate upon normal vascular endothelial surfaces. Once the endothelium has been broken, however, the deposition of platelets at the injury site has been observed repeatedly. It has been established that collagen is the principal substance in the subendothelium to which platelets adhere (1), although some recent studies indicate that platelets may also adhere to non-collagen substances located in the basement membrane (2).

---

*From the Division of Hematology, Roosevelt Hospital, New York, New York.

Following their adhesion to collagen, platelets release ADP (adenosine diphosphate) (3) and this adenine nucleotide, by a mechanism which is still disputed, produces changes in the platelets which result in their aggregation (4). In addition to ADP, collagen also induces the release of ATP (adenosine triphosphate), serotonin and other substances, and this process has been called the platelet "release reaction" (5).

Since the formation of a platelet aggregate appears to be an important early stage in the evolution of an arterial thrombus, it is possible that drugs which inhibit platelet aggregation may also prevent the formation of arterial thrombi. More pertinent to this discussion, they may also prevent the formation of platelet aggregates which may play a role in transient cerebral ischemic attacks.

As I shall describe shortly, aspirin appears to inhibit the release of platelet ADP and hence, by inhibiting ADP release, inhibits collagen-induced platelet aggregation. Since the latter is also important in the primary arrest of bleeding, it might be anticipated that aspirin ingestion produces a mild bleeding tendency. This finding in fact, was, reported in the 1950's by the French investigators, Beaumont (6) and Blatrix (7), who observed that aspirin in relatively small doses resulted in a prolongation of bleeding time. They also noted that this effect on the bleeding time was exaggerated in patients who had underlying bleeding disorders. These observations by the French investigators were little known in this country until their confirmation by Quick in the 1960's (8). Dr. Quick also made the important, additional observation that, unlike aspirin, sodium salicylate had no effect on the bleeding time (8), which indicated that the acetyl radical was somehow important in producing the mild defect in hemostasis after aspirin ingestion. Since platelet aggregation plays an important role in the primary arrest of bleeding, it seemed to us that aspirin might impede this process by interfering with platelet aggregation, and our first study in 1967 was designed to test this hypothesis.

In this study (9), we gave ten normal volunteers three grams of aspirin a day, for two and a quarter days. The study was conducted over a six-week period and, during the study, each subject received both the aspirin and, at a different time, a similar appearing lactose placebo.

Platelet aggregation was studied by an optical method in which platelet-rich plasma (PRP) is placed in a cuvette and the light which is transmitted through the cuvette is automatically recorded. The addition of an agent which causes platelet aggregation results in the formation of large platelet aggregates; this in turn allows more light to be transmitted through the cuvette and platelet aggregation is then recorded as an increase in the percent of light transmission. If, for example, one adds ADP to the PRP of normal subjects, the immediate formation of platelet aggregates results in an abrupt increase in percent of transmission. With collagen, platelet aggregation is also observed, but only after a short lag period during which ADP is released from the platelets. As mentioned earlier, it is this ADP released from the platelets by collagen which is directly responsible for their aggregation. Our studies confirmed the previous observations that the bleeding time became prolonged after aspirin ingestion. The mean bleeding time in the normal subjects was five minutes longer after ingesting aspirin than it was after ingesting the placebo. The studies also showed that this prolongation of the bleeding time was associated with a significant impairment in collagen-induced platelet aggregation. By contrast, aspirin ingestion did not inhibit ADP -induced aggregation. Since the platelets were still capable of responding to exogenously added ADP in a normal manner, the findings suggested that aspirin prevented collagen-induced aggregation by inhibiting the release of *endogenous* platelet ADP. Further studies showed this to be the case. Following aspirin ingestion, collagen-induced platelet ADP release was significantly reduced when compared with values obtained after ingesting a placebo.

The next study (10) which we performed was undertaken to investigate some of the possible mechanisms whereby aspirin inhibited platelet aggregation and ADP release. We used a somewhat smaller dose of aspirin. In the first study, subjects received ten tablets, or three grams a day for two and a quarter days; whereas in the second study they were given a single one and a half grams dose (5 tablets), and the effect on the bleeding time and on platelets were studied two hours after ingestion. In addition to using a different dose, we also studied the effect of sodium salicylate. For our hypothesis concerning the mechanism of aspirin to be correct, sodium salicylate should have little effect on platelets since Quick reported that this drug did not prolong the bleeding time (8).

In this second study, six normal subjects received either aspirin, sodium salicylate, or a placebo, at different times over an eight-week period. As in the previous study, the bleeding time was slightly increased after aspirin ingestion, when compared with the values obtained after ingesting a placebo. As reported by Quick, sodium salicylate had no effect on the bleeding time. Similar to the results obtained in our first study, aspirin ingest resulted in impaired collagen-induced aggregation; and, by contrast, sodium salicylate had no effect. Similarly, we found that aspirin inhibited the amount of ADP released from platelets by collagen, whereas sodium salicylate had no effect. These differences between aspirin and sodium salicylate were also observed when the drugs were added to PRP *in vitro.*

There are other types of agents which can cause platelets to aggregate. For example, if epinephrine is added to platelet-rich plasma at 37°, one observes two waves of aggregation. The first wave is due to the effect of epinephrine itself; the second wave is caused by the release of intrinsic platelet ADP (11). If one adds aspirin to PRP, one observes that the first wave of platelet aggregation occurs in a perfectly normal manner, whereas, the second wave of platelet aggregation, which is due to ADP release, is completely abolished. These studies again demonstrate that aspirin inhibits platelet ADP release and, by so doing, abolishes the second wave of epinephrine-induced aggregation. When sodium salicylate, rather than aspirin, was added to the PRP, both the first and second waves of platelet aggregation occurred quite normally. The effects of aspirin in abolishing the second (as opposed to the primary) wave of ADP -induced aggregation will be discussed later by Dr. Zucker.

In another experiment, we compared the effects of different concentrations of aspirin in inhibiting collagen-induced platelet ADP release. The studies were performed by incubating PRP with aspirin and then measuring the amount of ADP released from the platelets after stirring the mixture with collagen. With 0.05 mM of aspirin, a marked and significant decrease in platelet ADP release was obtained. Increasing the concentration to 0.5 mM produced a slightly greater inhibitory effect, but no further degree of inhibition was obtained when concentrations in excess of 0.5 mM were used.

From my readings of the literature, I would expect that a blood concentration of 0.5 mM of aspirin could be easily achieved by ingesting two to four standard aspirin tablets (12). Since a significant effect on platelets was obtained with a concentration of .05 mM, one can see that the oral dose of aspirin required to inhibit platelets is small indeed. With sodium salicylate, little or no inhibitory effect was observed at any concentration. We also performed this experiment using different concentrations of connective tissue and found that, for each concentration of aspirin, the inhibitory effect could be overcome to some extent with higher concentrations of connective tissue. However, for all the concentrations of connective tissue which were used, a maximal inhibitory effect was achieved with 0.5 mM of aspirin increasing the concentration above this did not result in enhanced inhibition.

As I indicated earlier, collagen induces the release from platelets of other substances, such as ATP and serotonin, and we performed experiments to see whether the inhibitory effects of aspirin were specific for ADP release. We found, *in vitro* experiments, that aspirin inhibited the collagen-induced release of platelet ATP as well. Dr. Zucker has also shown that aspirin also inhibits the release of platelet serotonin (13). The conclusions to be reached from all these experiments is that aspirin inhibits the entire platelet-release reaction.

The mechanism whereby aspirin inhibits the release reaction is not entirely clear at present, but the effects of aspirin appear to occur very rapidly and are of long duration. The duration of the aspirin-induced defect in ADP release was determined in two normal subjects (10) after obtaining base-line studies. They ingested a single 1.5 gram dose of aspirin, and collagen-induced platelet ADP release was subsequently studied. Two hours after the dose, ADP release was markedly decreased and remained decreased after 6 and 24 hours. Blood salicylate concentration was determined, and the maximum values of salicylate were obtained 6 hours after the dose. It should be emphasized that this was measuring salicylate, and not acetyl salicylic acid, which is hydrolized very rapidly in the blood.

At the end of 24 hours, there was no detectable salicylate in the blood; nonetheless, platelet ADP release was still markedly diminished and remained so on the second and third day after aspirin ingestion. Pre-treatment values were not obtained until the fourth to seventh day. Since the platelet life span is approximately seven to ten days, the studies suggest that aspirin results in irreversible damage to all the platelets present in the blood, and that the detectable effect of aspirin on the platelet population probably does not disappear until the affected platelets have been replaced by a population of new platelets.

To summarize, aspirin, unlike sodium salicylate, inhibits the release of platelet ADP and, as a consequence, results in the impairment of collagen-induced platelet aggregation. Aspirin also inhibits the secondary wave of epinephrine-induced platelet aggregation by a similar mechanism. These findings may explain the mild hemostatic defect produced by aspirin which would indicate that it should be avoided in patients with bleeding disorders and where control of hemostasis may be a problem.

A more intriguing outcome of these studies is the possibility that, by inhibiting platelet aggregation, aspirin may be a useful anti-thrombotic agent. As Dr. Evans will describe later, there is a very good evidence that the formation of a platelet aggregate plays an important role in the evolution of an arterial thrombus (14). This aggregate may form on collagen fibers which are exposed after the intima has been broken. If aspirin is capable of inhibiting collagen-induced platelet aggregation, may it also prevent arterial thrombus formation?

In the next experiments (15), performed with Drs. Callisto Danese and Choudary Voleti, we developed an experimental model of arterial thrombosis and studied the possible effect of aspirin in preventing the formation of thrombi. Both carotid and both femoral arteries of dogs were exposed and isolated between clamps. An endarterectomy was performed on the right-sided vessels and the blood flow was then re-established. The left-sided vessels were injured by instilling 0.1N H_2SO_4 into the segments for two minutes. Two days later the animal was sacrificed and the vessels were examined for the presence of thrombosis.

In preliminary studies, we found that lesions of this type produced total occlusion in about 30% to 50% of the vessels. We found that endarterectomy removed not only the intima and internal elastic membrane, but usually a significant amount of the media, as well. The chemical lesion resulted in much more extensive lesion. In addition to complete removal of the intima, we found fragmentation of the internal elastic membrane, and relatively severe degenerative changes in the media, as well.

We next studied the effects of drugs on thrombus formation. In this study, the dogs received a daily dose of either a lactose placebo, 300 mg of aspirin, or 200 mg of dipyridamole (persantine), another drug which has been used in an attempt to prevent thrombi. The animals treated were given these drugs for two days, and on the third day the vessels were injured by endarterectomy or H_2SO_4. The drugs were continued for two more days, and on the third day the animals were sacrificed and the vessels examined for the presence of thrombosis. The amount of thrombosis present in the segments were estimated either visually or, in some cases, by flow studies. The results showed that treatment with aspirin reduced the incidence of complete occlusion in the endarterectomized vessels from 42% to 11%, while the incidence in the acid-treated segments was reduced from 29% to 2%. In a second study, it reduced the incidence of acid-induced thrombosis from 39% to 0%. In contrast to the effects of aspirin, dipyridamole had no effect in preventing thrombosis.

In summary, then, we began with the earlier observations of the French investigators that aspirin prolongs the bleeding time and concluded from recent studies that this may result from the inhibitory effect of aspirin on platelet aggregation. We proceeded to explore the possibility that aspirin might, as a consequence of its effect on platelets, be a useful anti-thrombotic agent; and the results with our particular animal model would appear to support this possibility. Can this widely used drug, by preventing platelet aggregates from forming in extracranial arteries, also prevent some types of transient cerebral ischemic attacks? In the final analysis, of course, these questions can only be answered by clinical trials, which I hope this group will shortly undertake.

REFERENCES

1. Hugues, J., and Lapiere, C.M.: Nouvelles recherches sur l'accolement des plaquettes aux fibres de collagene. *Thromb. Diath. Haemorrhag.*, *11*:327, 1964.
2. Baumgartner, H., and Spaet, T.: Personal communication.
3. Hovig, T.: Release of platelet aggregating substance (adenosine diphosphate) from rabbit blood platelets induced by saline "extract" of tendons. *Thromb. et Diath. Haemorrhag.*, *19*:264, 1963.
4. Gaarder, A., Jonsen, J., Laland, S., Hellem, A., and Owren, P.A.: Adenosine diphosphate in red cells as factor in platelet adhesiveness. *Nature, 192:531*, 1961.
5. Holmsen, H., Day, H.J., and Stormorken, H.: The blood platelet release reaction. *Sc. J. Haemat., Suppl. 8.*, 1969.
6. Beaumont, J.L., Caen, J., and Bernard, J.: Influence de l'acide acetyl salicylique dans les maladies hemorragiques. *Sang.*, *27*:243, 1956.
7. Blatrix, C.: Allongement du temps de saignement sous l'influence de certain medicaments. *Nouv. Rev. Franc Hemat.*, *3*:346, 1963.
8. Quick, A.J.: Salicylates and bleeding: the aspirin tolerance test. *Amer. J. Med. Sci.*, *252*:265, 1967.
9. Weiss, H.J., and Aledort, L.M.: Impaired platelet-connective tissue reaction in man after aspirin ingestion. *Lancet*, *1*:495, 1967.
10. Weiss, H.J., Aledort, L.M., and Kochwa, S.: The effect of salicylates on the hemostatic properties of platelets in man. *J. Clin. Invest.*, *47*:2169, 1968.
11. MacMillan, D.C.: Secondary clumping effect in human citrated platelet rich plasma produced by adenosine diphosphate and adrenaline. *Nature*, *211*:140, 1966.
12. Levy, G., and Leonards, J.R.: Absorption, metabolism and excretion of salicylates. *In, The Salicylates, a Critical Biographical Review*. M. J. H. Smith and P. K. Smith, editors. Interscience Publishers, Inc., New York, 5, 1966.
13. Zucker, M.B., and Peterson, J.: Inhibition of adenosine diphosphate-induced secondary aggregation and other platelet functions by acetylsalicylic acid ingestion. *Proc. Soc. Exptl. Biol. Med.*, *127*:547, 1968.
14. Glynn, M.F., Murphy, E.A., and Mustard, J.F.: Platelets and thrombosis. *Ann. Intern. Med.*, *64*:715, 1966.
15. Weiss, H.J., Danese, C.A., and Voleti, C.D.: Prevention of experimentally induced arterial thrombosis by aspirin. *Fed. Proc.*, *29*:381, 1970.

Chapter VII

THROMBOEMBOLISM

GEOFFREY EVANS, M.B., JAMES F. MUSTARD, M.D.,
and MARIAN A. PACKHAM, Ph.D.

The majority of middle-aged persons in the Western World die from a cardiovascular disorder. A prominent factor in the morbidity and death from cardiovascular disorders is thromboembolism (1). Myocardial infarction, many strokes, some renal disease and much peripheral vascular disease are almost invaribly associated with diseased arteries. A high proportion of these diseased arteries are affected by mural and occlusive thrombi that play a significant part in causing dysfunction of the effected organ (2,3,4).

During the past twenty years, numerous attempts have been made to institute measures for the management of thromboembolic disorders. One of these forms of therapy has been the use of anticoagulants, designed to prevent or reduce fibrin formation. This therapy has proved effective for the management of venous thromboembolism, particularly during the post-operative period, and in complications associated with pregnancy (5,6). Anticoagulant drugs, however, have not produced any significant effect on the overall morbidity and mortality from the complications of arterial disease, such as myocardial infarction and strokes (7,8,9). Assuming that thrombosis is involved in the death of patients with vascular disease who die from strokes or myocardial infarction, this evidence indicates that drugs such as dicoumarol are relatively ineffective in the management of arterial thrombosis. These clinical findings are not incompatible with what we now know about the formation of thrombi. Venous thrombi have a large coagulation component and, therefore, should be susceptible to the action of orally administered anticoagulants. In contrast, thrombi that form on the arterial side have a smaller coagulation component and, therefore, may be less susceptible to the action of such anticoagulants. These drugs are also relatively ineffective in prolonging the duration of patency of femoral popliteal bypass grafts, and reducing the embolic complications of cardiac prosthetic valves (10,11).

The enthusiasm with which anticoagulant therapy was adopted for the treatment of arterial thrombosis indicates that the differences between arterial and venous thrombi were not taken into consideration. This is curious because investigators such as Bizzozero (12), Eberth and Schimmelbusch (13), and Welch (14) in the 1880's clearly demonstrated that arterial thrombi were initially composed of aggregated platelets and were not blood clots. Hence the rationale behind the use of anticoagulant drugs to prevent the initial accumulation of the platelet mass, which is the primary event in the formation of arterial thrombi, is open to serious question.

The knowledge acquired during the past ten years reinforces the initial observations of the investigators in the 1880's and indicates that we do have new approaches to the diagnosis and management of thromboembolic disease, particularly arterial thromboembolism. These observations also indicate that the dimensions of thromboembolic disease are much greater than have been appreciated. We should consider some of the recent evidence related to blood platelets. The other components of the problem which are important and deserve consideration, such as the fibrinolytic mechanism and blood coagulation, will not be discussed.

THROMBOSIS

An arterial thrombosis from flowing blood is initially composed of aggregated platelets with some fibrin around the platelet aggregates (15). Thrombosis and hemostasis represent the same reactions, that is, the response of the blood to vessel wall injury, and as far as we can tell the mechanisms involved in each of these processes are the same (16). When a blood vessel is cut, a mass of aggregated platelets plugs the cut vessel within three to four minutes. This is the process of hemostasis. The platelet mass extends from the tissue at the margins of the cut vessel across the lumen, and fibrin forms around the periphery of the aggregated platelets.

The fact that the same mechanisms are involved in hemostasis and thrombosis poses a therapeutic dilemma. Can we inhibit thrombosis without altering hemostasis? The evidence indicates that we can. Blood responds not only to vessel wall injury but also to intravascular stimuli (17). A mass of loosely aggregated platelets can be formed in a kidney capillary by means of an intravascular stimulus. We may look upon the reaction by which platelets can be made to aggregate as a general response of the blood to injury. The injury or stimulus can involve exposure of the subendothelial tissues in the vessel wall or the occurrence in the circulation of materials that can aggregate platelets. Intravascular stimuli include antigen antibody complexes, viruses, bacteria, endotoxin, adrenalin, serotonin, thrombin, and trypsin (18).

PLATELET AGGREGATION

To understand the response of blood to injury, it is essential to understand the mechanism involved in the formation of platelet aggregates: 1) the release of platelet constituents initiated by connective tissue in the vessel wall or constituents in the blood such as antigen antibody complexes; 2) the adherence of platelets to each other, induced by adenosine diphosphate (ADP) which can be released from the platelets by the stimuli just listed or from other injured cells; and 3) the influence of blood coagulation on platelet aggregation and on the stabilization of these aggregates by the formation of fibrin (19).

PLATELET RELEASE REACTION

When platelets are exposed to collagen or other stimuli such as antigen antibody complexes, they adhere to it. In contrast to the effect of ADP, the stimuli cause a profound structural change in the platelets, associated with the release of some of the platelet constituents (20,21). The release reaction is associated with the discharge of serotonin, histamine and adenine nucleotides (ATP and ADP) from the osmiophilic storage granules present in the platelets (22,23,24). The mechanism involved seems to be similar to the stimulus--secretion coupling mechanism described for other granule discharge processes such as those of the adrenal medulla (25,26). The release reaction itself involves metabolic energy and divalent cations (27, 28), and is differentiated from the non-specific release of cell constituents that occur when platelets are lysed. Other factors released from platelets include enzymes such as beta-glucuronidase, acid phosphatase, and cathepsin (29,30,31). Also released is a factor which caused contraction of smooth muscle and increases vessel wall permeability (17,32). Recently it has been reported that platelets also contain elastase that can be released (33). Antigen antibody complexes can also cause the release of platelet constituents (34). Viruses and bacteria can cause platelet clumping; but it has not been established that they cause the same degree of release of platelet constituents, although *in vitro* it can be shown that they do cause release of platelet nucleotides and serotonin (17). Endotoxin caused platelet aggregation (35), but it is believed that this involves the process of immune adherence (18,36) as well as the release reaction (18).

Another dimension to the reaction of platelets with intravascular stimuli is that the platelets can phagocytose particulate matter such as antigen antibody complexes and viruses (37). Platelet phagocytosis of particulate matter resembles leucocyte phagocytosis of particulate matter in many ways.

THE ADHERENCE OF PLATELETS TO EACH OTHER

When platelets are exposed to ADP, they change from their characteristic disc-shape to a more rounded form with pseudopods. In the presence of calcium and motion, the altered platelets are then able to adhere to each other. This process can be studied *in vitro* by placing platelets in a suspending fluid. As the platelets aggregate, light transmission increases and can be recorded. Following platelet aggregation by ADP, deaggregation occurs and the platelets eventually return to their original disc-shape and again become responsive to ADP. There does not appear to be any evidence that ADP can cause irreversible aggregation either *in vivo* or invitro (18). It is possible that the apparent irreversible platelet aggregates induced by ADP *in vitro* are an antifact of the *in vitro* test system.

The mechanisms involved in ADP-induced platelet aggregation have not been established. However, it is known that divalent cations are required (38); calcium is essential for aggregation, and magnesium appears to be important in deaggregation (38,39).

Metabolic energy is involved, and if the platelets lack glucose or are unable to utilize it, they become unresponsive to ADP (22,40). In addition, the platelets contain a contractile protein that resembles actomyosin (41), and it is believed that this is important in the process of platelet aggregation and deaggregation (42). Recently cyclic AMP (adenosine monophosphate) has been involved in the process of platelet aggregation and deaggregation (43,44,45).

BLOOD COAGULATION AND PLATELET AGGREGATION

There appears to be a complex relationship between platelet aggregation and blood coagulation. When platelets are aggregated by ADP, the platelet phospholipoprotein at the membrane is exposed and accelerates the clotting reaction (46,47,48). This phospholipoprotein is involved in inter-actions between factors IX and VII and between factors X and V (50, 51)). Thrombin is generated in the area of the platelet aggregates at a rate faster than can be diluted by flowing blood and neutralized by antithrombin. The thrombin can cause the release of further platelet constitutes in the same manner as collagen and antigen antibody complexes (18, 24). Thrombin also causes the conversion of fibrinogen to fibrin, further accelerates the coagulation process (52, 53), and activates the fibrin stabilizing factor, factor XIII. These observations explain why the fibrin is interspersed only among the platelets at the surface of freshly formed thrombi or platelet aggregates seen in electronmicrographs (15, 55, 56).

OTHER FACTORS INFLUENCING PLATELET AGGREGATION

Epinephrine and norepinephrine can cause platelet aggregation (57,58). The mechanisms involved appear to be related in part, at least, to the release of platelet ADP (59,60). In addition, adrenalin potentiates the action of ADP and thrombin in causing platelets to aggregate (61,62,63). Adrenalin also accelerates blood coagulation (64). Serotonin is another platelet constituent that can be released and cause aggregation (57,65). Its effect, however, is transient compared to that of adrenalin.

INHIBITION OF PLATELET AGGREGATION

A variety of compounds have been described which inhibit

ADP-induced platelet aggregation. These compounds include the adenine compounds, prostoglandin E_1, methylzanthines, pyrimido-pyrimidine compounds, and a number of other compounds many of which are used as vasodilators such as nitroglycerine and intersain (18). In *in vitro* studies, prostoglandin E_1 has been found to be the most potent of the inhibitors of aggregation (66, 67), 2-chloroadenosine (68) has also been found to be extremely active, as has a derivative of AMP, 2-methyl thio-AMP (69). Since almost all of these compounds have also vasodilator effects, they have not proven to useful for *in vivo* inhibition of platelet aggregation (70).

INHIBITION OF THE PLATELET RELEASE REACTION

Many of the compounds that inhibit ADP-induced platelet aggregation will, in high concentrations, also inhibit the release of platelet constituents induced by stimuli such as collagen, or antigen-antibody complexes (18). In addition to these compounds, the non-steroidal anti-inflammatory drugs (71,72) and the imipramine type of compounds (59), inhibit the release reaction. These compounds differ from the others in that they do not inhibit ADP-induced platelet aggregation. Lipids influence this process, and it has been demonstrated that phosphatidylserines inhibit the platelet release reaction (34). When platelets are exposed to non-steroidal anti-inflammatory drugs such as acetylsalicylic acid (aspirin), and sulfinpyrazone, collagen-induced platelet aggregation is inhibited, and this is associated with diminished release of platelet constituents such as the adenine nucleotides and serotonin (71-72). It is believed that this inhibition of the release of platelet constituents prevents collagen-induced platelet aggregation. Not only is this true for collagen, but also for antigen-antibody complexes and low concentrations of thrombin (71,72).

THE *IN VIVO* EFFECT OF INHIBITION OF PLATELET AGGREGATION

As mentioned earlier, the formation of a hemostatic plug at the end of a cut vessel is a similar process to that involved in thrombosis. It is possible, therefore, to use the process of hemostasis to explain whether changing platelet function by the administration of compounds that inhibit platelet aggregation, the platelet release reaction, or a combination of both, influences the response of the blood to vessel injury. The administration to rabbits of drugs in doses that inhibit the reaction of platelets with collagen or inhibit ADP-induced platelet aggregation, leads to a significant prolongation of the total bleeding time (72). These findings probably explain several well known clinical observations. Aspirin has been known for years to be associated with gastrointestinal bleeding (74). Although it has effects on the mucosa of the gastrointestinal tract it is apparent that the inhibition of platelet function could be a contributing factor to the bleeding seen with compound.

Another complication of these non-steroidal anti-inflammatory drugs is their effect on the development of spontaneous hemorrhage in subjects receiving oral anti-coagulant therapy (75). It was observed in rabbits that dicoumarol or phenylbutazone, in doses that alone did not alter the primary and total bleeding time, did cause marked impairment of hemostasis when given together in such doses (19). In these circumstances, two of the three primary mechanisms in hemostasis were altered, that is, the reaction of platelets with collagen or basement membrane, or both, and the ability of blood to generate thrombin for the blood coagulation reaction. Thus, partial inhibition of two of the three mechanisms involved in the response of blood to injury leads to a severe impairment of hemostasis. For similar reasons, the administration of aspirin to a hemophiliac leads to a severe impairment of hemostasis.

Heparin is of interest in this respect, because it is not only an anticoagulant but, when given in higher doses, can also inhibit the platelet response to collagen and to ADP (77). When heparin is given in doses that are conventionally used for an anticoagulant effect, it has only a slight effect on hemostasis. However, when it is given in higher doses that influence platelet function as well, it severely impairs hemostasis (19).

Another method by which these inhibitory compounds can be studied is in extracorporeal shunts. These shunts provide a surface in which blood interacts as it does with prosthetic materials. In these experiments, the shunt contains a bifurcation that is connected to the carotid artery and jugular vein of the experimental animal. Aspirin and phenylbutazone significantly decrease the amount of deposit formed on the bifurcation of the shunts

(71,72,79). In other experiments with rabbits, prior administration of acetylsalicylic acid was shown to reduce the incidence of occlusive femoral vein thrombosis produced by local injection of sodium morrhuate (79).

Three of the compounds that inhibit the platelet release reaction or platelet aggregation are known to be active in man. Dipyridamole reduces the incidence of thromboembolism in patients with prosthetic heart valves (80) and inhibits platelet aggregation (81). Aspirin prolongs the bleeding time in man (82) and prolongs platelet survival (83). Aspirin has a property that the other non-steroidal anti-inflammatory drugs do not appear to have; that is, the effect of a single dose of aspirin may last for several days (84). This may or may not be a beneficial effect, depending upon the circumstances. Sulfinpyrazone is one of the more interesting compounds. It was the material used initially to observe the effects of these drugs on platelets in man (85).

The effectiveness of these compounds in man is perhaps best demonstrated by their action on the rejection episodes that occur in transplanted human kidneys. The rejection episodes are associated with anuria and the accumulation of large masses of platelets in the renal vessels (86, 87), This work has been developed largely by Mowbray (87) and Porter (88) and confirmed in other experiments, particularly in experimental animals (88). Study of the behaviour of (51) Cr-labeled platelets in these individuals has demonstrated accumulation of the radioactivity over the transplanted kidney during a rejection episode. If, at this time, compounds that inhibit platelet aggregation are administered, the radioactive platelets leave the kidney and return to the circulation. Renal function is restored. The platelets that return to the circulation appear to have the same survival time as that of platelets from patients not undergoing a rejection episode. These studies indicate that in the early stages thrombi are in a balance between formation and dissolution. If the balance is tilted in favor of dissolution, the mass disappears.

RESPONSE OF BLOOD TO INJURY IN DISTURBANCES OF THE MICRO-CIRCULATION

The concept of thrombosis is mainly centered around the process in large vessels. However, the mechanisms involved in the response of blood to injury (18) indicate that intravascular aggregates may be formed and have a significant effect on the microcirculation.

The intravenous infusion of antigen-antibody complexes into rabbits causes a formation of platelet aggregates in the pulmonary vessels (32). This is associated with a fall in the arterial pressure and a rise in the venous pressure. This change has usually been attributed to antigen-antibody complex aggregates blocking the pulmonary circulation (89). However, if the animals are treated with non-steroidal anti-inflammatory drugs, such as aspirin and sulfinpyrazone, the fall in the platelet count caused by the infusion of the antigen-antibody complex can be prevented (32). When rabbits are treated in this manner, there is no fall in the arterial pressure or rise in the venous pressure associated with the infusion of antigen-antibody complexes. Furthermore, histological examination of the lung fails to reveal platelet aggregates in the pulmonary bed. Thus, if platelet aggregation by antigen-antibody complexes is inhibited, the fall in the arterial pressure and rise in venous pressure are prevented. It appears therefore, that the blood pressure changes seen in the anaphylactic response to the intravenous infusion of antigen-antibody complexes are at least initially related to platelet aggregation and not just to trapping antigen-antibody complexes in the pulmonary circulation.

The intravenous infusion of endotoxin is known to be associated with fall of the arterial pressure and rise of venous pressure with the development of shock in rabbits (90). If rabbits are treated with drugs such as sulfinpyrazone, phenylbutazone, acetylsalicylic acid, or sodium salicylate before the intravenous infusion of the endotoxin, the platelet count does not fall and the blood pressure is maintained (32,91). Histological examination of the treated animals show that the endotoxin does not cause platelet aggregation in the pulmonary bed, such as is seen in the untreated animals. Following its infusion, endotoxin becomes associated with the platelets in the circulation (35,92). It is clear that prevention of this endotoxin inter-action with platelets protects the animals from the acute effects of the endotoxin infusion.

One of the consequences of repeated stimulation of the blood with endotoxin is the formation of fibrin deposits in the kidney giving rise to the generalized Schwartzman reaction (93). It appears that one mechanism of formation of this fibrin deposit is through the action of endotoxin on platelets. It is recognized that endotoxin can also accelerate blood coagulation (93), and that blood coagulation could initiate the formation of fibrin deposits in the kidney. If rabbits given endotoxin are treated with non-steroidal anti-inflammatory drugs, the renal lesions characteristic of the generalized Schwartzman reaction can be prevented (32,91). These observations indicate that the acute vascular syndromes associated with bacterial infection may be altered by the use of compounds that inhibit platelet aggregation. The studies also indicate that the response of blood to injury is a wider subject than just the effects of occlusive thrombi in large veins and arteries.

THE FATE OF THROMBI

In our understanding of the response of blood to injury, the resolution and organization of thrombi are also important. It was recognized early that an initial platelet-rich mass rapidly transformed to a mass of fibrin (14). More detailed studies have shown that at one hour the thrombus is composed of aggregated platelets surrounded by fibrin (15). By 24 hours, the platelets have been replaced by fibrin. In this process, the platelets separate from each other, plasma seeps in between the platelets, and clotting occurs. The platelets disintegrate so that the picture at 24 hours is of a mass of fibrin with platelet debris interspersed among the fibrin fibers. The thrombus material is rapidly invaded by polymorphonucleocytes, and by 24 hours mononuclear cells are present. By 11 days, a thrombus of this type is organized into a lesion full of young, smooth muscle cells and connective tissue and covered with endothelium. It is important to emphasize that a transformed platelet thrombus of 24 hours does not have the appearance of a blood clot. The age of an arterial thrombus obviously will influence the type of therapy that should be used to cause its dissolution.

REFERENCES

1. Kagan, A.: Information on thrombosis as a cause of death, from studies promoted by the World Health Organization. In *Thrombosis*, edited by S. Sherry, K.M. Brinkhous, E. Genton, *et al.* Washington, D. C., National Academy of Sciences, 1969, p. 236.

2. Mitchell, J.P.A., and Schwartz, C.J.: *Arterial Disease.* Oxford, Blackwell, 1965.
3. Moore, S., and Mersereau, W.A.: Micro-embolic renal ischemia and hypertension. *Canad, and M.A. J., 92:221*, 1965.
4. Gunning, A.J., Pickering, G.W., Robb-Smith, A.H.T., *et al:* Mural thrombosis of the internal carotid artery and subsequent embolism. *Quart. J. Med., 33:*155, 1964.
5. Sevitt, S.: Venous thrombosis and pulmonary embolism: Their prevention by oral anticoagulants. *Amer. J. Med., 33*:703, 1962.
6. Bottomley, J.E., Lloyd, O., and Chalmers, D.G.: Postoperative prophylactic anticoagulants in gynecology: A ten-year study. *Lancet, 2*:835, 1964.
7. Hilden, I., Iversen, K., Raaschou, F., *et al:* Anticoagulants in acute myocardial infarction. *Lancet, 2*:327, 1961.
8. Douglas, A.S.: Anticoagulant therapy in coronary artery disease. In *Thrombosis,* edited by S. Sherry, K.M. Brinkhous, E. Genton, *et al.* Washington, D. C. National Academy of Sciences, 1969, p. 690.
9. Marshall, J.: The role of anticoagulant therapy in the management of cerebrovascular disease. In *Anticoagulants and Fibrinolysins,* edited by R.L. MacMillan and J.F. Mustard. Philadelphia, Lea and Febiger, 1961, p. 305.
10. Evans, G., and Irvine, W.T.: Long-term arterial graft patency in relation to platelet adhesiveness, biochemical factors and anticoagulant therapy. *Lancet, 2*:353, 1966.
11. Genton, E.: Use of anticoagulants in the prevention of embolization from prosthetic heart valves. In *Thrombosis,* edited by S. Sherry, K.M. Brinkhous, E. Genton, *et al.* Washington, D.C., National Academy of Sciences, 1961. p. 708.
12. Bizzozero, J.: Ueber einen neuen Formbestrandtheil des Boutes und dessen Rolle bei der Thrombose und der Blutgerinnung. *Virchow Arch. Path. Anat., 90*:261, 1888.
13. Eberth, J.C., and Schimmelbusch, C.: *Die Thrombose nach Versuchen u. Leichenbefunden.* Stuttgart, Germany, Ferdinand Enke, 1888.
14. Welch, W.H.: The structure of white thrombi. *Trans. Path. Soc., Philadelphia, 13*:281, 1887.
15. Jorgensen, L., Rowsell, H.C., Hovig, T., et al: Resolution and organization of platelet-rich mural thrombi in carotid arteries of swine. *Amer. J. Path., 51*:681,1967.
16. Mustard, J.F.: Hemostasis and thrombosis. *Seminars Hemat., 5*:91, 1969.
17. Packham, M.A., Nishizawa, E.E., and Mustard, J.F.: Response of platelets to tissue injury. In *Biochem. Pharmacol. Suppl.* Pergamon Press, London, Oxford, 1968. p. 171.
18. Mustard, J.F., and Packham, M.A.: Factors influencing platelet function: Adhesion, release and aggregation. *Pharmacol. Rev., 22,* No. 2 p. 97-187.
19. Mustard, J.F., and Packham, M.A.: The biochemistry of primary hemostasis. Plenary Session Paper. XII Congress of the International Society of Hematology, New York, 1968, p. 306.
20. Hovig, T.: Release of a platelet aggregating substance (adenosine diphosphate) from rabbit blood platelets induced by saline "extract" of

tendons. *Thromb. Diath. Haemorrh.*, *9*:264, 1963.

21. Spaet, T.H., and Zucker, M.B.: Mechanism of platelet plug formation and role of adenosine diphosphate. *Amer. J. Physiol.*, *206*:1297, 1964.
22. Bak, I.J., Hassler, R., May, B., *et al.*: Morphological and biochemical studies on the storage of serotonin and histamine in blood platelets of the rabbit. *Life Sci.*, *6*:1133, 1967.
23. Tranzer, J.P., Da Prada, M., and Pletscher, A.: Electron microscopic study of the storage site of 5-hydroxytryptamine in blood platelets. *Advances Pharmacol*, *6* (part A): 125, 1968.
24. Holmsen, H., Day, H.J., and Stormorken, H.: The blood platelet release reaction. *Scand. J. Haemat.*, *Suppl. 8*:1, 1969.
25. Stormorken, H.: The release reaction of secretion: A general basic phenomenon related to phagocytosis/pinocytosis. *Scand. J. Haemat. Suppl.*, *9*:1, 1969.
26. Douglas, W.W.: Stimulus-secretion coupling: The concept and clues from chromaffin and other cells. *Brit. J. Pharmacol.*, *34*:451, 1968.
27. Muer, E.H., Hellem, A.J., and Rozenberg, M.C.: Energy metabolism and platelet function. *Scand. J. Clin. Lab. Invest.*, *19*:280, 1967.
28. Kinlough, R.L., and Mustard, J.F.: Unpublished observations.
29. Marcus, A.J., Zucker-Franklin, D., Safier, *L.B.*, *et al.*: Studies on human platelet granules and membranes. *J. Clin. Invest.*, *45*:14, 1966.
30. Day, H.J., Holmsen, H., and Hovig, T.: Subcellular particles of human platelets: A biochemical and electron-microscopic study with particular reference to the influence of fractionation techniques. *Scand. J. Haemat.*, *Suppl.*, *7*:1, 1969.
31. Giudici, G., and Turazza, G.: Activités lysosomiques des plaquettes du sang humain. *Hemostase*, *4*:91, 1964.
32. Mustard, J.F., Evans, G., Packham, M.A., *et al.*: The platelet in intravascular immunological reactions. In *Cellular and Humoral Mechanisms in Anaphylaxis and Allergy*, edited by H.Z. Movat, Basel, S. Karger, 1969, p. 151.
33. Robert, B., Legrand, Y., Pignaud, G., *et al.*: Activité elastinolytique associée aux plaquettes sanguines. *Path-Biol.* (Paris), *17*:615, 1969.
34. Movat, H.Z., Mustard, J.F., Taichman, N.S., *et al.*: Platelet aggregation and release of ADP, serotonin and histamine associated with phagocytosis of antigen-antibody complexes. *Proc. Soc. Exp. Biol. Med.*, *120*:232, 1965.
35. Howowitz, H.I., Des Prez, R.M., and Hook, E.W.: Effects of bacterial endotoxin on rabbit platelets: 11. Enhancement of platelet factor 3 activity in vitro and in vivo. *J. Exp. Med.*, *116*:619, 1962.
36. Spielvogel, A.R.: An ultrastructural study of the mechanisms of platelet-endotoxin interaction. *J. Exp. Med.*, *126*:235, 1967.
37. Mustard, J.F., and Packham, M.A.: Platelet phagocytosis. *Series Haemat.* *1,2*:168, 1968.
38. Born, G.V.R., and Cross, M.J.: Effects of inorganic ions and of plasma proteins on the aggregation of blood platelets by adenosine diphosphate. *J. Physiol.* *170:*397, 1968.
39. Ardlie, N.G., Packham, M.A., and Mustard, J.F.: Adenosine diphosphate-induced platelet aggregation in suspensions of washed rabbit platelets. *Brit. J. Haemat.*, In press, 1970.

40. Kinlough, R.L., Packham, M.A., and Mustard, J.F.: Glucose and platelet aggregation (Abstr) *Fed. Proc., 28*: 509, 1969.
41. Bettex-Galland, M., and Luscher, E.F.: Thrombosthenin--acontractile protein from thrombocytes: Extraction from human blood platelets and some of its properties. *Biochim. Biophys. Acta., 49*:536, 1961.
42. Davey, M.G., and Luscher, E.F.: Biochemical aspects of platelet function and hemostasis. *Seminars Hemat., 5*:5, 1968.
43. Wolfe, S.M., and Shulman, N.R.: Adenyl cyclase activity in human platelets. *Biochem. Biophys. Res. Commun., 35*:265, 1969.
44. Zieve, P.D., and Greenough, W.B. III: Adenyl cyclase in human platelets: Activity and responsiveness. *Biochem. Biophys. Res. Commun., 35*, 1969.
45. Salzman, E.W., and Neri, L.L.: Cyclic 3',5'-adenosine monophosphate in human blood platelets. *Nature, 224*:609, 1969.
46. Mustard, J.F., Hegardt, B., Rowsell, H.C., *et al:* Effect of adenosine nucleotides on platelet aggregation and clotting time. *J. Lab. Clin. Med., 64*:548, 1964.
47. Castaldi, P.A., Larrieu, M.J., and Caen, J.: Availability of platelet factor 3 and activation of factor XII in thrombasthenia. *Nature, 207*:422, 1965.
48. Hardisty, R.M., and Hutton, R.A.: Platelet aggregation and the availability of Platelet factor 3. *Brit. J. Haemat., 12*:764, 1966.
49. Marcus, A.J.: The role of lipids in blood coagulation. In *Advances in Lipid Research,* edited by R. Paoletti, D. Kritchevsky. New York, Academic Press 1966, p. 1.
50. Hemker, H.C., and Kann, M.J.P.: Reaction sequence of blood coagulation. *Nature, 215*:1201, 1967.
51. Esnouf, M.P.: Biochemical aspects of blood coagulation. Plenary Session Paper, XII Congress of the International Society of Hematology. New York 1968, p. 315.
52. Nachman, R.L.: Platelet proteins. *Seminars Hemat., 5*:18, 1968.
53. Rapaport, S.I., Schiffman, S., Patch, M.J., *et al.:* The importance of activation of antihemophilic globulin and proaccelerin by traces of thrombin in the generation of intrinsic prothrombinase activity. *Blood, 21*:221, 1963.
54. Ozge-Anwar, A.H., Connell, G.E., and Mustard, J.F.: The activation of factor VIII by thrombin. *Blood, 26*:500, 1965.
56. Hovig, T.: The ultrastructure of blood platelets in normal and abnormal states. *Series Hemat. I., 2:3,* 1968.
57. Hovig, T., Rowsell, H.C., Dodds, W.J., *et al.:* Experimental hemostasis in normal dogs and dogs with congenital disorders of blood coagulation. *Blood, 30*:636, 1967.
58. Mitchell, J.R.A., and Sharp, A.A.: Platelet clumping in vitro. *Brit. J. Haemat., 10*:78, 1964.
59. Mills, D.C.B., Robb, I.A., and Roberts, G.C.K.: The release of nucleotides, 5-hydroxytryptamine and enzymes from human blood platelets during aggregation. *J. Physiol., 195*:715, 1968.
60. Haslam, R.J.: Role of adenosine diphosphate in the aggregation of human blood platelets by thrombin and by fatty acids. *Nature, 202*:765, 1964.
61. Mills, D.C.B., and Roberts, G.C.K.: Effects of adrenaline on human

blood platelets. *J. Physiol., 193*:443, 1967.
62. Ardlie, N.G., Glew, G., and Schwartz, C.J.: Influence of catecholamines on nucleotide-induced platelet aggregation. *Nature, 212*:415, 1966.
63. Thomas, D.P.: The role of platelet catecholamines in the aggregation of platelets by collagen and thrombin. In *Platelets in Hemostasis,* and *Exp. Biol. Med., 3*:129, Basel, S. Karger, 1968.
64. Ozge-Anwar, A.H., Rowsell, H.C. Downie, H.G., *et al.:* The effect of adrenaline infusions on blood coagulation in normal and haemophilia B dogs. *Thromb. Diath. Haemorrh., 15*:349, 1966.
65. Baumgartner, H.R., and Born, G.V.P.: Effects of 5-hydroxytryptamine on platelet aggregation. *Nature, 218*:137, 1968.
66. Emmons, P.R., Hampton, J.R., Harrison, M.J.G., *et al.:* Effect of prostaglandin E, on platelet behaviour in vitro and in vivo. *Brit. Med. J., 2*:468, 1967.
67. Kloeze, J.: Influence of prostaglandins on platelet adhesiveness and platelet aggregation. In *Proceedings of the 2nd Novel Symposium Stockholm,* June 1966, edited by S. Xergstrom, B. Samuelsson. Stockholm, Almqvist and Wiksell. New York, Interscience, 1967, p. 241.
68. Born, G.V.R.: Strong inhibition by 2-chloroadenosine of the aggregation of blood platelets by adenosine diphosphate. *Nature, 202*: 95, 1964.
69.,Michal, F., Maguire, M.H., and Gough, G.: 2-Methylthioadenosine-5'phosphate: A specific inhibitor of platelet aggregation. *Nature, 222*:1073, 1969.
70. Born, G.V.R., Haslam, R.J., Goldman, M., *et al.:* Comparative effectiveness of adenosine analogues as inhibitors of blood-platelet aggregation and as vasodilators in man. *Nature, 205*:678, 1965.
71. Packham, M.A., Warrior, E.S., Glynn, M.F., *et al.:* Alteration of the response of platelets to surface stimuli by pyrazole compounds. *J. Exp. Med., 126*:171, 1967.
72. Evans, G., Packham, M.A., Nishizawa, E.E., *et al.:* The effect of acetylsalicylic acid on platelet function. *J. Exp. Med., 128*:877, 1968.
73. Nishizawa, E.E., Hovig, T., Lotz, F., *et al.:* Effect of a natural phosphatidyl serine fraction on blood coagulation, platelet aggregation and haemostasis. *Brit. J. Haemat., 16:*487, 1969.
74. Gast, L.F.: Influence of aspirin on haemostatic parameters. *Ann. Rheum. Dis., 23*:500, 1964.
75. Olwin, J.H.: The choice of anticoagulant drugs--adequate anticoagulant therapy. In *Anticoagulants and Fibrinolysins,* edited by R.L. MacMillan, J.F.Mustard. Philadelphia, Lea and Febiger, 1961, p. 240.
76. Quick, A.J.: Bleeding time after aspirin ingestion. *Lancet, 2*:50, 1968.
77. Rowseil, H.C., Glynn, M.E., Mustard, J.F., *et al.:* Effect of heparin on platelet economy in dogs. *Amer. J. Physiol., 213*:915, 1967.
78. Evans, G., and Mustard, J.F.: Platelet surface reaction and thrombosis. *Surgery, 64*:273, 1968.
79. Peterson, J., and Zucker, M.B.: The effect of adenosine monophasphate, arcaine and anti-inflammatory agents on thrombosis and platelet function in rabbits. *Throm, et Diath. Haem. XXIII, 1*:148, 1970.
80. Sullivan, J.M., Harken, De, and Gorlin, R.: Effect of dipyridamole on the incidence of arterial emboli after cardiac valve replacement. *Circulation, 39 (suppl 1):* 1-149, 1969.

81. Emmons, P.R., Harrison, M.J.G., Honour, A.J., *et al.:* Effect of dipyridamole on human platelet behaviour. *Lancet, 2:*603, 1965. 1965.

82. Mielke, C.H. Jr., Kaneshiro, M.M., Maher, I.A., *et al.:* The standardized normal ivy bleeding time and its prolongation by aspirin. *Blood, 34*:204, 1969.

83. Evans, G., and Mustard, J.F.: Unpublished observations.

84. Weiss, H.J., Aledort, L.M., and Kochwa, S.: The effect of salicylates on the hemostatic properties of platelets in man. *J. Clin. Invest., 47*:2169,

85. Smythe, H.A., Ogryzlo, M.A., Murphy, E.A., et al: The effect of sulfinpyrazone (anturan) on platelet economy and blood coagulation in man. *Canad. M. A. J., 92:*1038, 1968.

86. Porter, K.A., Dossetor, J.B., Marchioro, T.L., *et al.:* Human renal transplants: 1.Glomerular changes. *Lab. Invest.,16*:153, 1967.

87. Mowbray, J.F.: Methods of suppression of immune responses. Proceedings of the IXth International Congress of Internal Medicine, *Excerpta Medica Int. Cong. Series 137*:106, 1966.

88. Lowenhaupt, R., and Nathan, P.: Platelet accumulation observed by electron microscopy in the early phase of renal allotransplant rejection. *Nature, 220*:822, 1968.

89. Austen, K.F.: Anaphylaxis: Systemic, local cutaneous and in vitro. In the *Inflammatory Process*, edited by BW Zweifach, L Grant, RT McCluskey. New York, Academic Press, 1965, p. 587.

90. Brockman, S.K., Thomas, C.S., and Vasko, J.S.: The effect of Escherichia coli endotoxin on the circulation. *Surg. Gynec. Obstet., 125*:763, 1967.

91. Evans, G., and Mustard, J.F.: Inhibition of the platelet-surface reaction in endotoxin shock and the generalized Schwartzman reaction. (Abstr) *J. Clin. Invest., 47*:31a, 1968.

92. Herion, J.C., Herring, W.B., Palmer, J.H., *et al.:* Cr^{51}-labeled endotoxin distribution in granulocytopenic animals. *Amer. J. Physiol., 206*:947, 1964.

93. McKay, D.G.: *Disseminated Intravascular Coagulation.* New York, Hoeber Medical Division, Harper & Row, 1965.

Chapter VIII

EFFECTS OF ASPIRIN AND OTHER ANTI-INFLAMMATORY AGENTS ON PLATELETS

MARJORIE B. ZUCKER, Ph.D.*

We have been interested in the release of platelet constituents induced by ADP and epinephrine as well as by connective tissue particles (CT). Figure 1 illustrates aggregation induced in human, citrated, platelet-rich plasma at 37°C by three concentrations of ADP. (Methods are described in detail elsewhere (1). A low concentration causes reversible aggregation. With a critical concentration of ADP, here 1 μM, aggregation occurs in two phases. The second wave is associated with release of ADP (2,3,4). This type of release is similar to the connective tissue-induced release reaction

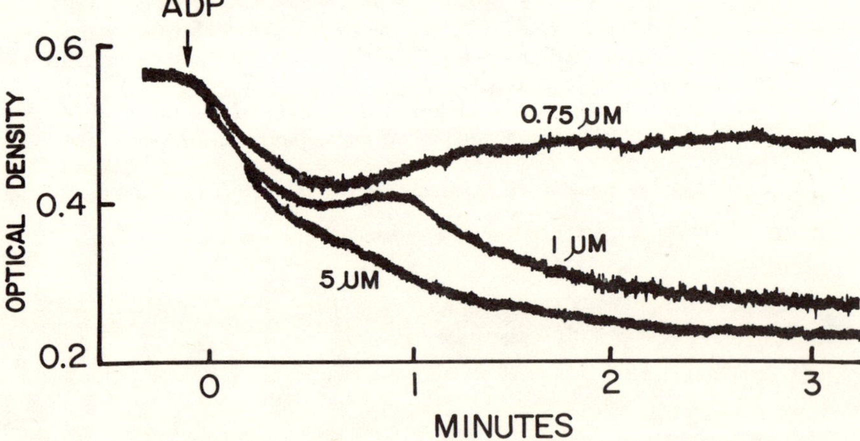

Figure 1. Aggregation of citrated human platelet-rich plasma induced by several concentrations of ADP.

*Partially supported by the American National Red Cross and grants from the National Heart Institute (HE-05003 and HE-12859). Contribution No. 212 from the Blood Research Laboratories, ANRC.

(5). It seems to be a surface reaction; the suspension must be stirred and the platelets must touch each other in order to release ADP (6). With a higher concentration of ADP, e.g., 5 μM, the two phases are merged and the aggregation curve is not biphasic.

The ADP-induced release reaction is characteristic of human platelets as well as of some, but not all, animal species (4). This type of release may provide a mechanism for a chain reaction, as Born pointed out some years ago (7). If platelets stick to the blood vessel wall, they release ADP and a few more platelets then adhere. But what makes more platelets stick to the second layer of platelets to form a solid hemostatic plug or thrombus head? Is it just the ADP from the original platelets which adhered to the wall, or do the platelets in the second layer release ADP, making more platelets adhere and release ADP, and so on?

Epinephrine produces a small first wave and a very pronounced second wave of aggregation (8). The second wave results from release of ADP from the platelets (2,3,4). Animal platelets do not show this reaction to epinephrine (4).

In some studies, only about 80% of normal subjects who have had no aspirin for several days showed a release reaction with ADP and epinephrine (6,9,10) but many laboratories now using an aggregometer routinely for clinical studies find that virtually all normal subjects not on aspirin show a second wave of aggregation with epinephrine or a critical concentration of ADP. The variables responsible for the failure of certain samples from certain subjects from certain laboratories to demonstrate release are not completely understood.

When the double wave occurs, not only is ADP released but also platelet factor 4 (an anti-heparin factor) (4,11,12,13) and ^{14}C-Serotonin (3,6,9,14) (if the platelets have been permitted to take up radioactive serotonin, which they do avidly).

We found that the release reaction induced by ADP is inhibited by ingestion of a relatively small amount of aspirin (6); others have shown that release induced by CT or epinephrine is also inhibited. More specifically, when aggregation is tested in blood drawn after aspirin ingestion, the response to the critical ADP concentration is no longer biphasic, but reversible (6). The response to high ADP concentrations is unchanged because release is not important in this response (6,9). With high as well as low concentrations of epinephrine, the second wave of aggregation is abolished (9,10,13,15,16,17), whereas with CT, inhibition of aggregation is more marked with low concentrations than with high (16). Inhibition of release by aspirin ingestion can also be detected by measuring release of platelet factor 4 induced by ADP or CT (12,13) and release of ^{14}C-serotonin induced by ADP (6,9,14), epinephrine (9), or CT (9).

Similar inhibition of aggregation (10,14,16,17) and release of platelet factor 4 (12,13) and ^{14}C-serotonin (14) are noted when aspirin is added to platelet-rich plasma *in vitro.* We have recently made extensive studies on the effect of aspirin *in vitro* (14), using the technique of ^{14}C-serotonin release because of its simplicity. The technique, described elsewhere (18,19), is essentially as follows:

Platelet-rich plasma is incubated for a few minutes with ^{14}C-serotonin (Nuclear Chicago Co., about 0.4 μM/liter and 0.016 μCi/ml final concentration). A 0.1 ml sample is taken for measuring total radioactivity in a liquid scintillation counter. Aliquots of 0.36 ml are placed in tubes. Isotonic saline (0.04 ml) is placed in one tube and a similar volume of CT, 100 μM ADP, or 500 μM epinephrine in others. The samples are shaken or inverted repeatedly for four minutes at 37° C. (ADP and epinephrine do not induce release at room temperature (19). They are then centrifuged and the radioactivity in 0.1 ml of each supernatant is measured. Usually the supernatant of the control sample contains less than 20% of the total radioactivity, the remainder having been taken up by the platelets. When the supernatant of the other samples contains a higher percentage of the added radioactivity, release has occurred. Although high concentration of thrombin and connective tissue particles can release as much as 90% of the platelet-bound serotonin, high concentrations of ADP and epinephrine rarely release more than 50%.

Figure 2 shows release of ^{14}C-serotonin induced by several concentrations of CT. The amount of ^{14}C-serotonin released varied with the CT concentration. With relatively high concentrations, aspirin only partially inhibited release. As Weiss *et al.* noted for release of ADP (16), aspirin has an all-or-none type of effect. The maximally effective concentration of aspirin in our studies was very low--10-35 μM--and higher concentrations failed

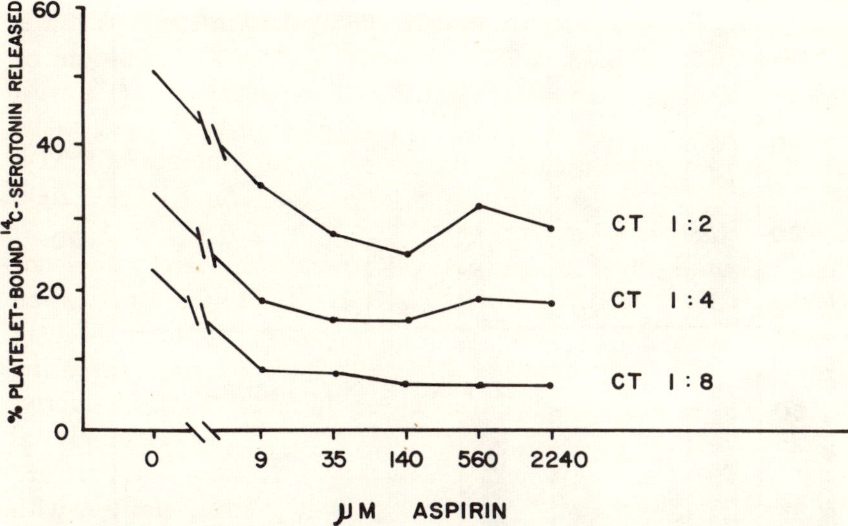

Figure 2. Effect of various concentrations of aspirin on the release of platelet-bound ^{14}C-serotonin induced by three different concentrations of connective tissue. (Reprinted by permission from *J. Lab. Clin. Med.*, Ref. 14).

to enhance inhibition. The inhibitory effect of aspirin is much enhanced by preincubating the drug at 37° C with platelet-rich plasma, as shown by O'Brien (10) and in Figure 3. Without preincubation, 640 μM aspirin was needed to inhibit either aggregation or ^{14}C-serotonin release. With a few minutes' preincubation, the required concentration was only 160 μM, and with 15-minute preincubation, 40 μM. This is the range of concentration that can be obtained in blood with low oral doses of aspirin (20). Probably Weiss *et al.* (16) found higher levels of aspirin necessary for maximal inhibition because they did not preincubate the platelets with the drug at 37° C. Figure 4 demonstrates that low concentrations of aspirin totally inhibit release induced by ADP and epinephrine.

Others have shown that the effect of a single, small oral dose of aspirin can last up to five days (10,15,16). If aspirin is to be useful as an antithrombotic agent it is also necessary to show that the platelets do not become tolerant of it--that is, that the impressive inhibitory effect on platelets persists for months when aspirin is ingested daily. According to a recent study carried out in this laboratory (9) on patients with rheumatic fever and rheumatoid

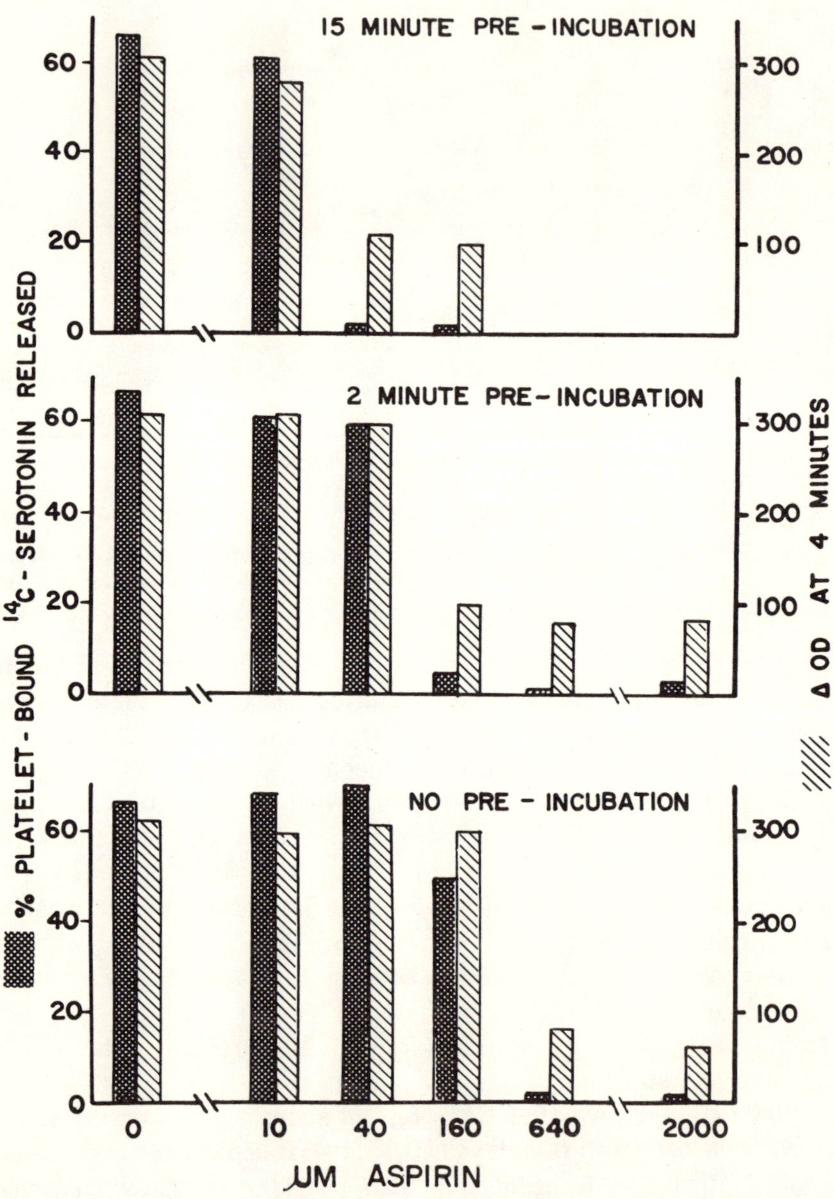

Figure 3. Effect of varying periods of aspirin incubation with platelet-rich plasma on the release of platelet bound ^{14}C-serotonin and the decrease in optical density induced by a suspension of connective tissue particles. (Reprinted by permission from *J. Lab. Clin. Med.*, Ref. 14.)

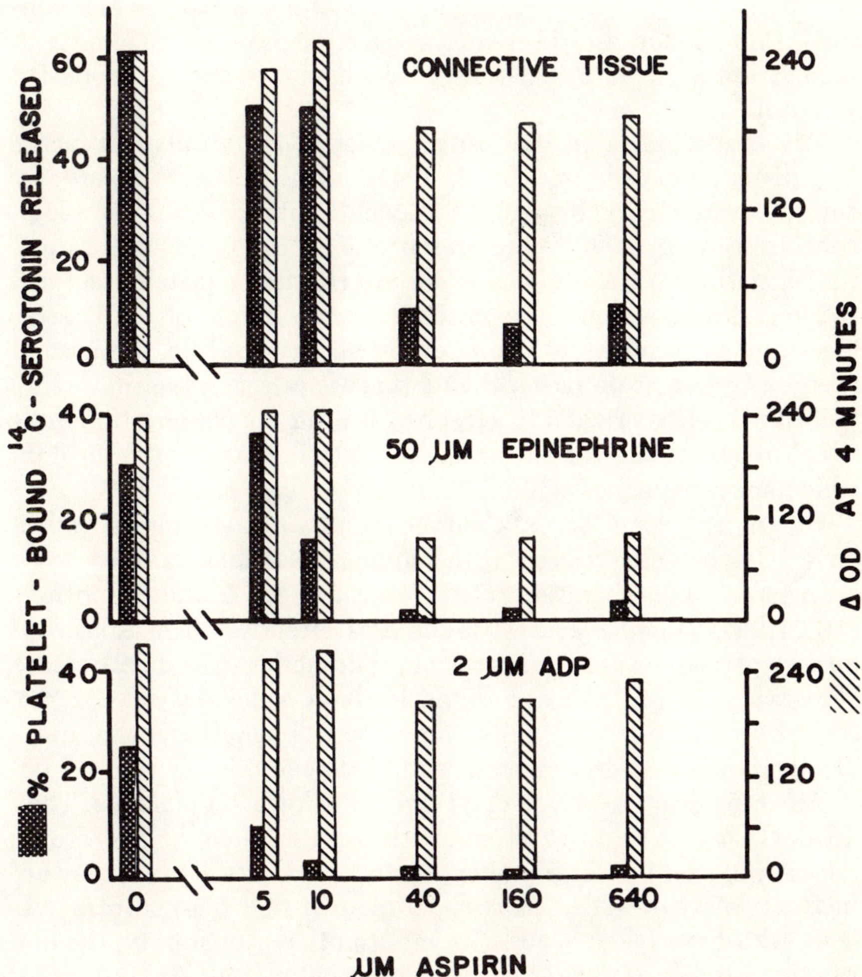

Figure 4. Effect of various concentrations of aspirin on the release of platelet-bound ^{14}C-serotonin and the decrease in optical density induced by a suspension of connective tissue particles, epinephrine, or ADP. (Reprinted by permission from *J. Lab. Clin. Med.*, Ref. 14.)

arthritis who have been taking aspirin for up to two years, its effect persists. Thus, none of the aspirin-takers had any release of ^{14}C-serotonin with 10 μM ADP or 50 μM epinephrine and CT-induced release was less marked than in subjects not on aspirin. The second wave of aggregation induced by epinephrine was absent, and aggregation induced by CT was less than in the controls. Control and aspirin-treated subjects showed no difference in aggregation induced by ADP because a high concentration of ADP was used.

This study indicated that aspirin failed to inhibit platelet factor 3 activity induced by 10 μM ADP. This activity apparently develops when marked aggregation occurs, either because of a high concentration of ADP in the presence of aspirin (9), or the critical concentration in the absence of aspirin (6). Little platelet factor 3 activity develops with the critical concentration of ADP after ingestion of aspirin (6), apparently because of the diminished degree of aggregation rather than a specific effect of aspirin.

Table 1 summarizes the effect of aspirin on platelet functions which relate to the formation of hemostatic plugs or the thrombi which are worrying us today.

We studied the effect of a number of other drugs besides aspirin on ^{14}C-Serotonin release from human platelets induced by a standard CT preparation (14) (Fig. 5). As found by others (16,21,22), salicylic acid is much less effective than aspirin on human platelets. In our experience, indomethacin is slightly more active than aspirin; O'Brien found it about equally active (21,22). Sulfinpyrazone was quite active and phenylbutazone quite inactive; the other drugs tested fell in between.

All these drugs seem to act at the same locus on platelets. They do not have an additive effect with aspirin when ^{14}C-serotonin release induced by CT is studied *in vitro,* and, like aspirin, they are ineffective when added *in vitro* to platelet-rich plasma from subjects who have taken aspirin by mouth (14). Apparently, the oral aspirin has already exerted a maximum effect. An important difference between the drugs, however, is their duration of action. O'Brien has shown that the effect of indomethacin lasts only a few hours, whereas that of aspirin and benorylate lasts for several days (22).

It should be emphasized that aspirin and the other drugs shown in Figure 5 have a very special effect on platelets. A number of other substances -- e.g., adenosine, and prostaglandin E1--inhibit ADP-induced primary aggregation and secondarily affect release. But aspirin, and other anti-inflammatory drugs do not affect primary aggregation by ADP and completely block ADP and

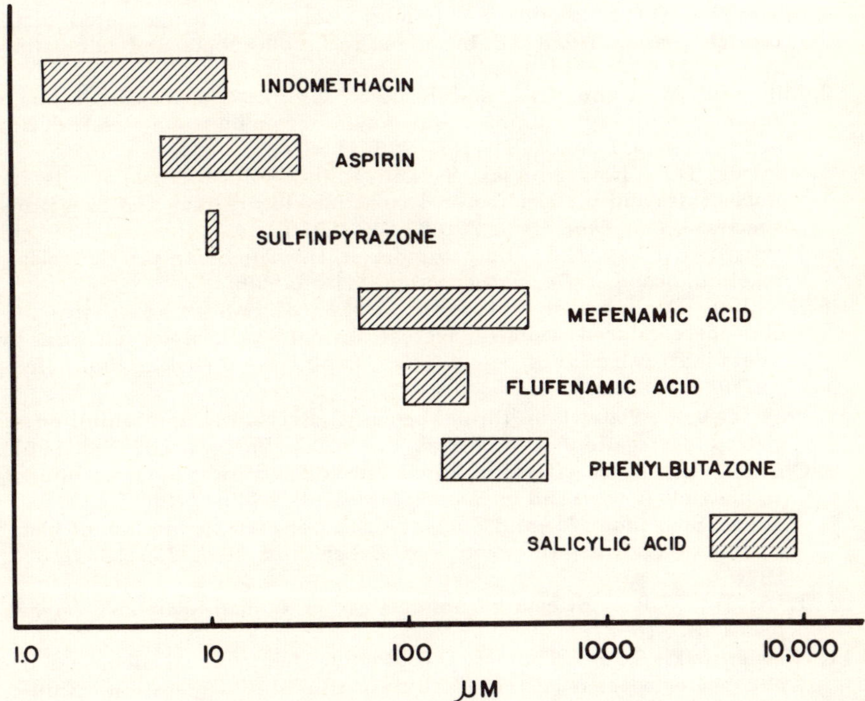

Figure 5. The concentrations of various anti-inflammatory drugs which cause 50% inhibition of ^{14}C-serotonin release induced by a suspension of connective tissue particles. (Reprinted by permission from *J. Lab. Clin. Med.*, Ref. 14.)

epinephrine-induced release.

In some experiments with rabbits we found that high doses of aspirin given intravenously inhibited thrombosis produced in femoral veins by sodium morrhuate (23). However, the doses were high, and the experiments may have little relevance to human material. I am not convinced that more animal experiments will lead us to useful conclusions and favor studies on thrombosis in man.

REFERENCES

1. Zucker, M.B.: Tests of platelet adhesion, aggregation and release, in Mammen E.F.; Anderson G.F.; Barnhart M.I. (eds): *Platelet Adhesion and Aggregation in Thrombosis: Countermeasures.* Supplement to Thromb. Diath. Haemorr., F. K. Schattauer Verlag, Stuttgart. In press.

2. Macmillan, D.C.: Secondary clumping effect in human citrated platelet-rich plasma produced by adenosine diphosphate and adrenaline. *Nature, 211*:140-144, 1966.

3. Mills, D.C.B., Robb, I.A., and Roberts, G.C.K.: The release of nucleotides, 5-hydroxytryptamine and enzymes from human platelets during aggregation. *J. Physiol., 195*:715-729, 1968.

4. Thomas, D.P., Niewiarowski, S., and Ream, V.J.: Release of adenine nucleotides and platelet factor 4 from platelets of man and four other species. *J. Lab. Clin. Med., 75*:607-618, 1970.

5. Holmsen, H., Day, H.J., and Stormorken, H.: The blood platelet release reaction. *Scand. J. Haematol., Suppl. 8*:1-26, 1969.

6. Zucker, M.B., and Peterson, J.: Inhibition of adenosine diphosphate-induced secondary aggregation and other platelet functions by acetylsalicylic acid ingestion. *Proc. Soc. Exper. Biol. Med., 127*:547-551, 1968.

7. Born, G.V.R.: Platelets in thrombogenesis: Mechanism and inhibition of platelet aggregation. *Ann. Royal. Coll. Surg. Eng., 36*:200-206, 1965.

8. O'Brien, J.R.: Some effects of adrenaline and anti-adrenaline compounds on platelets *in vitro* and *in vivo. Nature, 200*:763-764, 1963.

9. Atac, A., Spagnuolo, M., and Zucker, M.B.: Long-term inhibition of platelet functions by aspirin. *Proc. Soc. Exper. Biol. Med., 133*:1331-1333, 1970.

10. O'Brien, J.R.: Effects of salicylates on human platelets. *Lancet, 1*:779-783, 1968.

11. Niewiarowski, S., and Thomas, D.P.: Platelet factor 4 and adenosine diphosphate release during human platelet aggregation. *Nature, 222*:1269-1270, 1969.

12. Youssef, A.H., and Barkhan, P.: Inhibition by aspirin of release of antiheparin activity from human platelets. *Brit. Med. J., 3*:394-396, 1969.

13. O'Brien, J.R.: Platelet bound and soluble platelet factor 4: effects of aggregating agents, of aggregation and of aspirin. *Proc. Soc. Exper. Biol. Med.* In press.

14. Zucker, M.B., and Peterson, J.: Effect of acetylsalicylic acid, other nonsteroidal anti-inflammatory agents, and dipyridamole on human blood platelets. *J. Lab. Clin. Med., 76*:66-75, 1970.

15. O'Brien, J.R.: Aspirin and platelet aggregation. *Lancet, 1*:204-205, 1968.

16. Weiss, H.J., Aledort, L.M., and Kochwa, S.: The effect of salicylates on the hemostatic properties of platelets in man. *J. Clin. Invest., 47*:2169-2180, 1968.

17. Sahud, M.A., and Aggeler, P.M.: Platelet dysfunction--differentiation of a newly recognized primary type from that produced by aspirin. *New. Eng. J. Med., 280*:453-459, 1969.

18. Jerushalmy, Z., and Zucker, M.B.: Some effects of fibrinogen degradation products (FDP) on blood platelets. *Thromb. Diath. Haemorrh., 15*:413-419, 1966.

19. Valdorf-Hansen, J.F., and Zucker, M.B.: Effect of temperature and inhibitors on ^{14}C-serotonin release from human platelets. *Amer. J. Physiol.* In press.

20. Cotty, V., Zurzola, F., Beezley, T., and Rogers, A.: Blood levels of aspirin following the ingestion of commercial aspirin-containing tablets by

humans. *J. Pharm. Sci.*, *54*:868-870, 1965.

21. O'Brien, J.R.: Effect of anti-inflammatory agents on platelets. *Lancet*, *1*:894-895, 1968.
22. O'Brien, J.R., Finch, W., Clark, E.: A comparison of an effect of difference of anti-inflammatory drugs on human platelets. *J. Clin. Path.*, *23*:522, 1970.
23. Peterson, J., and Zucker, M.B.: The effect of adenosine monophosphate, arcaine and anti-inflammatory agents on thrombosis and platelet function in rabbits. *Throm. Diath. Haemorrh.*, *23*:148-158, 1970.

Table 1

EFFECT OF ASPIRIN ON PLATELET FUNCTIONS INVOLVED IN HEMOSTASIS AND THROMBOSIS

Test	*Inhibition with Aspirin*
Adhesion to Collagen and Sub-endothelial Fibers	Uncertain
Thrombin-induced Aggregation and Release	Slight
Collagen-induced Aggregation and Release*	Partial, dependent on CT concentration
ADP-induced Primary Aggregation	None
ADP-induced Secondary Aggregation and Release*	Complete
Epinephrine-induced Secondary Aggregation and Release*	Complete
Platelet Factor 3 Development	None
Platelet Retention in Glass Bead Column	None

*Release of platelet ADP, probably ATP (5), ^{14}C-serotonin and platelet factor 4.

Chapter IX

SOME ASPECTS OF PLATELET BIOCHEMISTRY*

AARON J. MARCUS, M.D.

Using a subcellular approach, our primary interest in human platelets has been to ascertain how they interact with such surfaces as blood vessel walls, and the proteins and lipoproteins found in the circulating blood (1). For example, what is it about the platelet membrane that permits its interaction with a blood vessel wall when its continuity is interrupted or when it is damaged? Leukocyte and erythrocyte membranes do not seem to take part in these early interactions. As yet, there are no answers to these questions. Despite intensive studies on the lipids of platelets (2), many platelet enzymes and proteins (3), we have come up with nothing that is biochemically unique to platelets and that might offer even a partial explanation of why such interactions occur.

Platelet membranes have been isolated in our laboratory and have been studied morphologically by Dr. Dorothea Zucker-Franklin in order to ascertain whether they are structurally different from other cell membranes. Was the classical bimolecular leaflet present? Was one portion of the leaflet larger than the other? Unfortunately, there is nothing that distinguishes the platelet membrane from a morphological standpoint. One interesting observation is that even on an osmium-fixed platelet, a good deal of material sticks to the outer leaflet--so-called "osmiophilic tags." When other fixatives became available for the study of platelet morphology, these tags were just a small portion of what adheres to the platelet membrane.

---

*From the Hematology Section, New York Veterans Administration Hospital, and the Department of Medicine, Cornell University Medical College. Supported by grants from the National Institutes of Health (HE 09070-07), the Veterans Administration, and the New York Heart Association.

Dr. Olav Behnke of Copenhagen has demonstrated that platelets have what he terms a "surface coat"--which he calls an "area of interest" in platelet function (4). This coat is not acquired when the platelet is in the circulation; it originates in the megakaryocyte as the platelet is developing. This emphasizes another problem in platelet research: When platelets are studied from the subcellular point of view, the surface coat is lost during manipulations required to prepare the platelet organelles. Furthermore, there is very little information on this surface coat, except that it does contain large amounts of glycoprotein and mucopolysaccharide material. One of the platelet compounds we are now studying, the gangliosides, may be structurally connected to the surface coat(5).

Platelet cytoplasm contains, as you probably know, several types of intracellular granules. Each one of these granules has its own membrane (6). Thus, the granule is probably a separate organelle, functioning independently. Some of these "granules" are actually mitochondria. The others are of several varieties. One has an eccentric body which we call a "bull's eye." Another has a homogeneous interior and is called an "alpha granule." These are characteristic of the kind of particle isolated when we prepare platelet membranes for study. Their reactivity in coagulation, enzyme content and lipid composition have been investigated in some detail. The membrane preparation is not pure plasma membrane because it contains membranes from intracellular organelles that have been distrupted in the homogenization and separation procedures. It also contains granules from smooth endoplasmic reticulum. Platelets do not have rough endoplasmic reticulum; they have little or no DNA.

We have arbitrarily designated a group of platelet "compartments" that we have studied with the subcellular approach. These are isolated by ultra-centrifugation on a sucrose gradient (1). The lowest compartment consists of intracellular granules and mitochondria. Further compartmentalization of the granule fraction is visible, but we have not as yet studied it. These granule fractions have several types of enzyme activity, some of which I shall summarize shortly. Lysosomal activity is prominent in the granules. At the top of the gradient, there is a band which consists of the plasma and intracellular membranes.

Thus, we have arbitrarily set up an admittedly artificial subcellular compartmentalization of platelets--i.e., a granule compartment, a membrane compartment, and a compartment that "floats" on top of the sucrose gradient (the soluble compartment). The soluble compartment is difficult to study because material may be present that originated in other fractions but was disrupted by homogenization. The enzymes and metabolic substances that have been found in these compartments comprise an ever-expanding list. Some platelet functions can be at least partially explained by the presence of these enzymes (6).

We have recently become interested in a group of glycolipids known as gangliosides. They have been found mainly in brain tissue and in several extraneural organs such as the adrenal medulla, where they seem to be present in cell membranes and in areas concerned with hormonal secretion (7). These glycolipids characteristically contain neuraminic acid. In platelets, about 0.6% of the lipid fraction is ganglioside, and it contains all of the lipid-bound neuraminic (sialic) acid. Studies on gangliosides in other tissues have suggested to us that this fraction could be an important site on the platelet membrane for biological interactions. As an example, Woolley's group has shown that the membrane receptor for serotonin in the brain is a ganglioside (8). By coincidence, this is one of the three main gangliosides found in platelets.

Other interesting functions have been attributed to gangliosides. For example, on some cell membranes the calcium-binding site has been postulated to be ganglioside (9). Recently, Brady's group at the NIH showed that ganglioside synthesis is altered after transformation of a cultured cell into a malignant growth phase (10).

These compounds may also be involved in the "excitability" of cell membranes. It has further been shown that the gangliosides in cell membranes of the central nervous system could be the site of binding of tetanus toxin (11). With such experiments in mind, we are now working on platelet gangliosides.

Positioning of this large molecule in the platelet membrane might help explain some of the biological activities in which platelets have been implicated. This molecule contains a long-chain fatty acid, as well as the amino alcohol, sphingosine. The fork-like structure of the molecule has been postulated by some to be jutting into the milieu of the cell, and it may serve as a "reactive site." The neuraminic acid is also a potentially active membrane site.

Recently we took part in an aspirin (ASA) study in collaboration with Dr. Al-Mondhiry and Dr. Spaet (12). Initially, they tried to determine whether aspirin was bound to platelets. The investigation produced some interesting results, but for reasons I will shortly mention, definite conclusions cannot be drawn.

We first took two forms of radioactive aspirin--ASA tagged in the carboxyl group, and then ASA tagged in the acetyl group. The question was: Did one or both groups attach to or enter the platelet? Incubation of platelets with these two forms of ASA yielded the following results: Al-Mondhiry demonstrated that the radioactive acetyl group was taken up by platelets, whereas the tagged carboxyl group was not. The inference was that platelets were nonspecifically combining with ASA and were in some way taking up the acetyl group from the aspirin. Deykin has shown that platelets can incorporate acetate into the lipids of their membranes and granules (13).

Therefore, were we merely studying nonspecific acetate incorporation by platelets? Unfortunately, it is still impossible to answer this question. What we *can* partially explain is why the aspirin effect lasts for four or five days.

When we incubated platelets with the acetyl-labeled aspirin and then prepared subcellular fractions, we could find radioactivity in comparable amounts in washed granules and membranes. The soluble fraction, which was also radioactive, was, of course, hard to evaluate because we may have destroyed granules and membranes when we prepared our homogenate. It was a bit perplexing to find that all compartments had taken up the label. However, this might be partially explained by results recently obtained by Zilversmit's group at Cornell. They have shown that some cells contain an enzyme which distributes lipids equally among all of the subcellular compartments.

There is yet another problem: Since we know that aspirin acetylates such proteins in the body as plasma proteins, was this merely a nonspecific acetylation process? If aspirin is added to platelets, or if a subject ingests ASA, the second wave of platelet aggregation is abolished. If acetic anhydride (a nonspecific acetylating agent) is added instead, the same effect is produced as with aspirin (12).

Thus, three important problems remain: 1) Did our results represent nonspecific acetylation? 2) Was it a case of acetate incorporation and nothing more? 3) Were the findings related to the interference of platelet function that occurs with aspirin? Unfortunately, our experiments did not permit conclusive answers to these questions.

In summary, then, we endeavored to gain insight into the nature of the interaction bewteen aspirin and platelet membranes and granules. We could show only that if platelets were incubated with aspirin tagged in the acetyl group, radioactivity could subsequently be detected in the platelets. What we cannot explain is whether this tagging was merely a nonspecific artifact of the incubation. There are two possibilities: nonspecific acetylation or acetate incorporation into lipid. Are these related in any way to the defect observed when aspirin is in contact with platelets--that is, the loss of second wave due to release of ADP?

Finally, I should like to leave you with the thought that an understanding of the mechanism of occlusive vascular disease, and ultimately its prevention, may be forthcoming from the further investigation of platelet biochemistry and physiology.

REFERENCES

1. Marcus, A.J., Zucker-Franklin, D., Safier, L.B.: *et al.:* Studies on human platelet granules and membranes. *J. Clin. Invest., 45*:14-28, 1966.
2. Marcus, A.J., Ullman, H.L., and Safier, L.B.: Lipid composition of subcellular particles of human blood platelets. *J. Lipid. Res., 10*:108-114, 1969.
3. Nachman, R.L., Marcus, A.J., and Safier, L.B.: Platelet thrombosthenin: subcellular localization and function. *J. Clin. Invest., 46*:1380-1389, 1967.
4. Behnke, Q.: Electron microscopical observations on the surface coating of human blood platelets. *J. Ultrastruct. Res., 24*:51-69, 1968.
5. Marcus, A.J., Ullman, H.L., Safier, L.B., *et al.:* Studies on human platelet gangliosides. *Fed. Proc., 29*:315, 1970.
6. Marcus, A.J., and Zucker, M.B.: *The Physiology of Blood Platelets: Recent Biochemical, Morphologic and Clinical Research.* New York, Grune, 1965.
7. Ledeen, R., Salsman, K., and Cabrera, M.: Gangliosides of bovine adrenal medulla. *Biochemistry,7*:2287-2295, 1968.
8. Woolley, D.W., and Gommi, B.W.: Serotonin receptors, VII. Activities of various pure gangliosides as the receptors. *Proc. Nat. Acad. Sci., 53*:959-963, 1965.
9. Lehninger, A.L.: The neuronal membrane. *Proc. Nat. Acad. Sci., 60*:1069-1080, 1960.

10. Brady, R.O., Borek, C., and Bradley, R.M.: Composition and synthesis of gangliosides in rat hepatocyte and hepatoma cell lines. *J. Biol. Chem.*, *244*:6552-6554, 1969.
11. Van Heyningen, W.E.: The fixation of tetanus toxin, strychnine, serotonin and other substances by ganglioside. *J. Gen. Microbiol.*, *31*:375-387, 1963.
12. Al-Mondhiry, H., Marcus, A.J., and Spaet, T.H.: On the mechanism of platelet function inhibition by acetylsalicylic acid. *Proc. Soc. Exp. Biol. Med.*, *133*:632-636, 1970.
13. Deykin, D., and Desser, R.K.: Incorporation of acetate and palmitate into lipids by human platelets. *J. Clin. Invest.*, *47*:1590-1602, 1968.
14. Wirtz, K.W.A., and Zilversmit, D.B.: Exchange of phospholipids between liver mitochondria and microsomes *in vitro*. *J. Biol. Chem.*, *243*:3596-3602, 1968.

DISCUSSION OF CHAPTERS VI THROUGH IX

Dr. Anthony P. Fletcher, St. Louis, Mo.: I think we have had a rare treat thus far, with some excellent papers. However, before opening the discussion, I would like to call on Dr. Zucker for some additional information regarding studies in progress.

Dr. Zucker: Dr. Edwin Salzman, a surgeon at Beth Israel Hospital in Boston, has given me permission to mention that he has been involved in testing the effect of aspirin on the incidence of venous thrombosis and pulmonary embolism in cup arthoroplasties of the hip. He and his colleagues felt they could not use an untreated group as a control because the incidence was too high.[1,2] They, therefore, compared other drugs to warfarin, previously shown to reduce the incidence of these complications Persantine (dipyridamole) was equivalent to no treatment. Dextran infusions--one a day at first, later cutting back to one every three days--were as effective as warfarin. Aspirin was somewhere between the efficacious dextran and warfarin, and the no-effect group. They are continuing this study. Their patients have venous thrombosis in which there is a large element of fibrin formation due to thrombin. In the sort of thrombi we are talking about here, where the platelet component is larger, we might expect a better effect from aspirin.

Dr. Fletcher: I think Dr. Sahud has somewhat similar data.

Dr. Mervyn A. Sahud, San Francisco, Calif.: I should like to demonstrate some similarities and differences between the effect of acetylsalicylic acid (ASA) and dipyridamole on platelets.

In an attempt to understand anti-platelet drugs, we have sought

---

[1] Salzman, E.W.; Harris, W.H.; and DeSanctis, R.W.: Anticoagulation for prevention of thromboembolism following fractures of the hip. *New Eng. J. Med., 275*:122-130, 1966.

[2] Salzman, E.W.: Venous thromboembolism in surgical patients. In Sherry, S.; Brinkhous, K.M.; Genton, E.; and Stengle, J.M. (eds): *Thrombosis.* Nat. Acad. Sci., Washington, D.C., 1969.

to characterize biochemical and physiological alterations induced in human platelets after ingestion of ASA (the prototype of non-steroidal anti-inflammatory agents) or dipyridamole. As might be expected from their divergent molecular structure, there are some striking differences. In fact, there appear to be more differences than similarities, so that it has become evident that neither drug is an ideal one, in and of itself.

The dipyridamole compounds have the ability to significantly impair platelet adhesiveness to glass, at least insofar as the Salzman technique is a function of this measurement. At 50 μg/ml, this drug can reduce platelet aggregation induced by small concentrations of adenosine diphosphate (ADP) added to an *in vitro* system of citrated platelet-rich plasma. However, its anti-aggregation properties are weak, and it does not significantly effect the bleeding time or the collagen-induced release reaction of platelets as measured in an *in vitro* system.

Theoretically, this compound appears to act in part by its inhibition of adenosine deaminase, thereby impairing breakdown of the adenosine base to inosine. Blockage of this enzyme system could then produce accumulation of adenosine and adenosine monophosphate, both of which are potent inhibitors of platelet aggregation. Although these compounds are cleared rapidly, they may be effective in local areas of stasis.

The impairment of platelet adhesiveness by the Salzman method can be demonstrated with as little as 100 mg. per day of dipyridamole and becomes increasingly more effective at 200, 300 and 400 mg per day. Particular attention must be paid to keeping the transit time of blood flow, that is, contact time of the blood flowing through the glass bead column, to 45 seconds per 5 ml. At 200 mg dipyridamole per day, we have seen a rise in platelet count which suggests some alteration in platelet production or utilization.

In summary, dipyridamole appears to be a well-tolerated agent which primarily impairs platelet adhesiveness, has weak anti-aggregant properties against adenosine diphosphate and metabolically effects the breakdown of adenosine to inosine by blockage of adenosine deaminase. The rise in platelet count that we have found in humans may reflect an alteration of platelet turnover. On the other hand, acetylsalicylic acid is a strong platelet antiaggregant because of its ability to impair the release of adenosine diphosphate from platelets after stimulation with collagen. In fact, the entire release reaction is impaired and release of platelet factors 3 and 4 are also blocked. This drug also prolongs the bleeding time and impairs platelet glycolysis.

Although the Salzman glass bead adhesiveness test seems to be a measure of both platelet-glass adhesion and platelet-aggregation, a depression in the adhesiveness test could not be demonstrated with ASA ingestion until a total dose of 2.4 gm per day had been taken, i.e., 16 tablets a day. During the waking hours, that would create a rather high salicylate concentration in the plasma and might produce symptoms of toxicity in some people. It is interesting that such large doses of ASA are needed to induce a defect in the adhesiveness index, when aggregation would appear in part to be a property measured by this test.

Acetylsalicylic acid did not create a rise in the platelet count such as dipyridamole did. Dr. Evans suggested that platelet survival was increased with aspirin usage. If platelet survival is increased, one would assume that there would have been some change in platelet count upwards, as occurs with dipyridamole. Perhaps there is a rapid feedback which reduces thrombopoiesis.

We have been studying the role of ascorbic acid in platelet metabolism. Prolonged administration of aspirin produces a distinct drop in the buffy coat concentration of ascorbic acid. Daniels, *et al.*, reported a study in 1934 demonstrating a rise in urine ascorbic acid in patients taking aspirin.[3] We have noted that uptake of ascorbic acid into platelets is impaired by acetylsalicylic acid but not sodium salicylate, and we think the mechanism responsible for ascorbic aciduria after aspirin ingestion is partly related to this impaired tissue uptake. Whether vitamin C plays a role in platelet function is unclear at this time.

Finally, I think it becomes apparent that these two drugs behave differently. Where dipyridamole may seem very weak in its ability to impair the release reaction, it seems to have a fairly potent effect on adhesion. I think it probably should not be entirely excluded from consideration, especially after hearing some

---

[3] Daniels, A.L., and Everson, G.J.: Influence of acetylsalicylic acid (aspirin) on urinary excretion of ascorbic acid. *Soc. Exp. Biol. & Med.*, *35*:20-24 (Oct.) 1936.

discouraging remarks at this conference about ASA. Perhaps there is a place where a combined therapy may be useful.

Dr. Fletcher: I should like to add a word about another trial of aspirin, that is to say, aspirin as a prophylactic in post-operative venous thromboembolism. This is the Medical Research Council clinical trial in England, which has been in progress for the past year and is, as yet, unpublished. It is a sophisticated trial, with thrombophlebitis being detected in post-operative patients using the I_{125} fibrinogen label method as the end point rather than thrombosis. This procedure demonstrates an approximately 30% incidence of thrombophlebitis in patients subjected to severe operations. Most of this thrombophletitis is clinically transient, lasting only 48 to 72 hours. The trial is of potentially great importance because extensive platelet studies have been performed on the patients by Dr. John O'Brien, and it is hoped we shall learn whether any of the conventional platelet function tests correlate with the subsequent development of thrombophlebitis. At the moment, with about 200 patients in the trial, which is still incomplete, I have been informed that no advantage has accrued to the aspirin-treated patients. However, as the trial proceeds, modified aspirin dosage schedules are being tested.

We have had some extremely interesting suggestions as to how aspirin might be used, and I would like to raise a specific point of significant practical importance. In view of the fact that aspirin is rapidly hydrolyzed--perhaps within half an hour of its absorption--and platelet turnover rates are high--ten to 15% a day--how often should aspirin be given to a patient to produce 100%, or near 100%, inhibition of secondary platelet release?

Dr. Zucker: I think perhaps each of us left this to the other person to emphasize, although Dr. Weiss did discuss it. The effect of two tablets of aspirin on platelets lasts for several days.

Dr. Fletcher: I do not think this is quite the point that I was trying to make. We know that platelets turn over extremely fast, so, to use a statistical term, we have distinct cohorts of platelets released. Now, is there any evidence that megakaryocytes are influenced by the action of aspirin; or is it conceivable that by giving a dose of aspirin you produce inhibition of circulating platelets and an hour later you have another cohort of platelets released? Does the post-aspirin cohort have normal functions?

Dr. Harvey J. Weiss, New York, N. Y.: I do not know the answer to that question, but I would assume that once the aspirin is hydrolyzed, and this occurs very rapidly, there is no further effect on circulating platelets. If you recall in one of the experiments I cited in my paper, aspirin inhibited platelet aggregation in citrated platelet-rich plasma for four to seven days after the ingestion of single 1.5 gm oral dose. Since this period corresponds to a period only somewhat less than the platelet life span, we assume that the effect of aspirin is to produce an irreversible defect in the circulating platelets. Platelet-rich plasma contains platelets of varying age, therefore, the net effect of a single dose of aspirin on this plasma would not disappear until the original population of platelets affected by the dose had been replaced by a new, unaffected population. While I do not know any direct evidence regarding the effect of aspirin on megakaryocytes, present evidence does not suggest that this is the case.

Dr. Fletcher: I would like to ask the people who presented papers thus far if there is a good way of approaching this problem experimentally?

Dr. Geoffrey Evans, Hamilton, Ont., Canada: Platelets are required in order to produce thrombosis. The question really is, then, how many platelets do you need to produce adequate hemostasis and thrombosis. In the experiments with endotoxin, we were unable to produce endotoxin shock if the platelet count was reduced to below about 20,000. In other experiments with shunts, again it was difficult to produce thrombosis in these extracorporeal shunts unless the platelet count was above 20,000 to 30,000.

The other important factor that we should consider is platelet turnover. We know that in certain conditions we have low platelet counts but adequate platelet turnover, and under these circumstances we do not get into any problems with hemostasis or thrombosis.

Dr. Fletcher: Now, would you attempt to answer one further question. If you were running a trial of aspirin as a prophylactic, how often would you think it would be necessary to give it per day, assuming it is hydrolyzed within half an hour to an hour?

Dr. Evans: Well, I would think that if one gives 5 grains of aspirin once or twice a day, it would certainly be adequate.

Dr. Fletcher: So you would think that if you gave aspirin once or twice a day you would have about 95% of the platelets permanently affected, and that would, in your view, be pharmacologically effective?

Dr. Truitt: I think it will become obvious, when we get to the metabolism of salicylates, that the effect you are talking about considerably outlasts the circulating unhydrolyzed aspirin or even, perhaps, the salicylate levels derived from aspirin.

Dr. Fletcher: The question at issue is one of optimal pharmacological effect at all times. Supposing a pharmacological regimen, at one instant of time, produces a situation in which 90% of circulating platelets are physiologically defective in a patient, i.e., the platelets failed to support thrombosis, but 10% of his platelets are newly released and physiologically competent, will this patient be protected either partially or wholly against thrombosis; or should we aim to devise pharmacological regimens which render virtually 100% of all circulating platelets defective at all times?

Dr. Truitt: Until you can decide how many platelets must be inhibited from aggregating in order to inhibit the entire process, you will not know. As a matter of fact, I was about to call aspirin a "hit-and-run drug." I believe Dr. B. B. Brodie at NIH introduced this term. This is where the action of the drug is essentially complete within a short time, but its effect far outlasts the duration of the drug at the site. The best example that Dr. Brodie used for this is of platelets affected by reserpine. In this instance, block of serotonin or catecholamine uptake by the platelets persists for several days after an initial dose of reserpine, although we know by radio-labeled studies that the tenure of reserpine is quite short compared with this effect. In the case in question here, it is interesting that aspirin has a prolonged action possibly as a result of transacetylation of proteins. This would be an easy explanation for this effect, if it works out.

Dr. Fletcher: I introduced this problem simply because of the obvious practical importance. If you are going to run a clinical trial, you should run it under the most efficient drug conditions, and I just wanted to establish whether anybody knew what they were.

Dr. Mark L. Dyken, Indianapolis, Ind.: Dr. Evans reported several clinical trials in patients with myocardial infarction and transient cerebral ischemic attacks with very good preliminary results. I wonder what the dosage was in those cases?

Dr. Evans: They were all given sulfinpyrazone, which is the agent I have been employing for inhibiting platelets. The other study which I mentioned was that of Tonks, in Cardiff; not my study. He has been using aspirin.

Dr. Dyken: Do you know the dosage?

Dr. Evans: I think it was two tablets twice a day, but I am not quite sure.

Dr. Fletcher: I think it was only one, actually. I talked with Dr. Tonks last year--he is a charming fellow--but he could not really tell me why he started this.

Dr. Evans: That's right. He has no idea.

Dr. Fletcher: It is absolutely fascinating. He just found it to be clinically useful.

Dr. Fields: I think at this point there is a bit of history that might be brought to your attention. When I was talking with Dr. Weiss on the telephone at the time I invited him to join us for this conference, he mentioned an interesting reference which he had found in an obscure medical journal. I hope that he will tell us about it. It is an apochryphal story that may be important as background information. The observations described are fascinating.

Dr. Weiss: About a year ago, I attended a meeting at which I proposed a study of aspirin as a possible prophylaxis against recurrent myocardial infarction. While riding to the airport after the meeting, a colleague mentioned a report on just this subject that he vaguely recalled reading in a regional medical journal about fifteen years earlier. Upon returning home I gave this fragmentary information to our very competent hospital librarian, who proceeded to find, within an hour, the article to which my colleague had undoubtedly referred. It was written by Dr. L. L. Craven of Glendale, California, and published in the *Mississippi Valley Medical Journal.*[4] The following day, a copy of the article arrived at my office.

Dr. Craven, I gathered, had practiced general medicine for over forty years. He reported on his use of aspirin in the prophylaxis of coronary and cerebral thrombosis during the previous ten years.

[4]Craven, L.L.: Prevention of coronary and cerebral thrombosis. *Miss. Valley Med. J.*, *78*:213, 1956.

His rationale for using aspirin was based on his previous observations that aspirin occasionally caused a mild bleeding tendency. He argued that since bleeding and thrombosis were, in a sense, opposite sides of the same coin, perhaps a drug which produced a mild bleeding tendency might also prevent thrombosis. He, therefore, prescribed two aspirin tablets a day to 8,000 men. His results, obtained over a period of seven to ten years, were stated in bold type, "Not a single case of detectable coronary or cerebral thrombosis occurred among patients who have faithfully adhered to this regimen." I would gather, however, that his use of two daily aspirin tablets as an anti-thrombotic agent was not greeted with wild acclaim by many of his colleagues. Dr. Craven conceded that he did not know why it worked, but argued that a similar statement could be made about quinine therapy for malaria and electric shock therapy in psychiatric disorders. he reiterated his intention to continue using aspirin as an anti-thrombotic agent.

Needless to say, Dr. Craven's study lacked proper controls. If, however, subsequent controlled studies confirm his findings and conclusions, I would nominate his observations as a masterpiece of clinical observations.

Dr. Fletcher: Don't forget Dr. Tonks. He made the same one. Dr. Hass, would you compare the virtues of dipyridamole with aspirin?

Dr. Hass: With regard to diapyridamole, a study was done in England[5] by Acheson, Danta, and Hutchinson--the same Hutchinson who, with Yates, did the elegant study of extracranial arterial disease, correlating it with post mortem findings in the brain. In 169 patients with ischemic cerebral vascular disease, they randomized the administration of dipyridamole. They had about 80 patients each in the treatment and control groups. The dipyridamole treatment group, for a period of fourteen months, received 400 milligrams a day. They did not, as in the case of Sullivan's study of thrombosis on prosthetic valves, also administer dicumarol. The dipyridamole treated group of patients, at the end of fourteen months, showed no discernible difference from the frank strokes. For the next eleven months, they increased the dose

[5]Acheson, J., Danta, G., and Hutchinson, E.C.: Controlled trial of dipyridamole in cerebral vascular disease. *Brit. Med. J.*, *1*:614-615, 1969.

controls in the recurrence of either transient ischemic attacks or to 800 mg. of dipyridamole a day, and again found no discernible difference in the residual treatment group from the controls in recurrence rates of transient ischemic attacks or of frank strokes. Their conclusion was that dipyridamole did not appear to affect the natural history of occlusive cerebrovascular disease over a 25-month period.

I will make one point about this study, which applies also to all other previous studies of stroke with the exception of the present surgical study of extracranial arterial disease. The investigators did not describe prospective angiographic studies of the cerebral vasculature in these patients. I think that this kind of prospective angiographic evaluation is terribly important to include in future studies where drugs are employed, or at least in one phase of a future drug trial. There may be another group of patients where angiography is not done, but certainly a core group should have angiography.

It is possible, I suspect--and perhaps Dr. Stallones can help us with this--that the 169 patients may have assorted themselves in such a way that ulcerated plaques, just on random distribution, fell more in one group of 85 than in another. In this kind of situation, one would be hard put to really evaluate the true meaning of the study described. It stands, however, as a negative study.

Dr. Fletcher: Dr. Evans, I would like to ask you to tell us about sulfinpyrazone because, in some ways, you made as big a claim as anybody for the clinical utility of this drug.

Dr. Evans: Sulfinpyrazone (Anturane) is a drug which has been used mainly for its uricosuric properties. It was perhaps the original drug which was noted to have anti-platelet surface properties. The dosage which we are using is 200 mg q.i.d., and we then assess platelet activity both in the glass bead columns and by testing platelet aggregation to collagen in the aggregometer. When we have adequate platelet suppression, we maintain the patient at this dosage.

Regarding any problems following administration of the drug, we have one case of allergy to sulfinpyrazone which ceased when the drug was stopped. However, it did not return when the drug was recommenced. We have had three to four patients who have complained of headache following administration of the drug, but these patients also complained of headache following administration of placebo. The evidence, therefore, from a study of 400 to 500 patients, is that we have had no major untoward reactions which we could show were due to the administration of the drug.

Dr. Thomas Kantor, New York, N. Y.: I want to point out that sulfinpyrazone is related to a metabolic product of butazolidin. I was wondering whether or not you know which one was the active form of the drug?

Dr. Evans: Are you worried about the white cell count?

Dr. Kantor: No, not at all. I am wondering whether butazolidin works because it is degradated into something like sulfinpyrazone.

Dr. Evans: I am sorry, but I do not know.

Dr. Hass: Dr. Evans, what was the average dose of sulfinpyrazone that you gave to your patients?

Dr. Evans: It was 800 mg to a gram a day.

Dr. Fletcher: you gave 250 mg four times a day, was that right?

Dr. Evans: Yes.

Dr. Sahud: I would like to get back once more to the question of dosage that you originally raised. I think it is true that when you give a very small dose, you get an effect which *in vitro* is quite remarkable. But, on the other hand, there are some limited dose dependency tests that have been performed. One is the simple bleeding time. You give a low dose of aspirin, which gives a very small prolongation of bleeding time--Dr. Weiss has shown this--and with a higher dose of aspirin, you get a longer extension of bleeding time. There is probably a limit to how long you can prolong the bleeding time after aspirin. There is also a limit to how much collagen you can use and overcome the reaction with the aspirin. Most people say a dose of between 35 and 50 millimolar *in vitro* concentration will completely inhibit the collagen-induced release of adenosine diphosphate. So there is a point to which you can raise the concentration of aspirin and still overcome its inhibition on platelets by increasing--doubling or tripling--the concentration of collagen. In other words, I am not quite sure that a small dose is necessarily as effective as a large dose.

In addition, as I mentioned before, it took up to sixteen tablets of aspirin before we could see a drop in the adhesiveness index in a normal person, using the Salzman technique. Although more studies obviously need to be done on drug dose relationship, there appear to be some reasons for giving a higher dose.

Dr. Ehrenfeld: Perhaps my remarks at the moment are preempting some of the later discussion, but I think this point should be borne in mind in our discussion of transient cerebral ischemic attacks and their prevention. It should be recognized that the results of surgery are quite good, specifically in the class of transient ischemic attacks related to the carotid artery. In fact, most surgical series report amelioration of symptoms well in excess of 90%, and in our own series, over 95%. Stroke prevention is similarly enhanced. The morbidity and mortality rates are less than two percent. I think we should bear this in mind when considering any other type of therapy.

Dr. Fields: I would agree with Dr. Ehrenfeld that the surgical treatment of carotid artery disease has produced some spectacular results in the hands of experienced surgeons; however, there is little or no evidence of stenosis, even though the radiologist may describe a roughened or ulcerated area in the wall of the vessel. It is to this latter group of cases that we should address our attention when considering the potential merits of a new form of medical therapy.

Dr. Frank Yatsu, San Francisco, Calif.: I would like to ask Dr. Evans, relevant to Dr. Hass' criticism of Hutchinson: What percentage of your patients had arteriographic evidence of an ulcerated lesion?

Dr. Evans: Although our patients had arteriographic studies, I cannot tell you exactly what percentage had ulcerated lesions.

Regarding the effect of aspirin on platelet retention in glass bead columns, we are measuring many factors in addition to platelets. We have found that it is extremely difficult to reduce the platelet retention in glass bead columns of normal patients by the administration of aspirin. however, if one studies this in patients with high platelet retention, then it is less difficult to reduce the level. Again, I think this reflects the large number of factors which come into play when we pass whole blood through glass bead columns. We are, on the one hand, measuring platelet activity--the effects of both platelet interaction with the surface and platelet interaction with other platelets. The fact that plasma is present and plasma is absorbed into the surface of the glass bed columns is also important in the interaction of whole blood with the glass bed columns.

Regarding the platelet interaction with the glass surface, we know that younger platelets interact, far more than the older platelets, with surfaces such as glass, antigen-antibody complexes, collagens, etc., and I think in some way we are measuring some form of platelet survival.

Dr. Fletcher: We will have to stop now. However, I should like to conclude by saying that I do not think we should forget anticoagulants completely because of our current enthusiasm for aspirin trials.

Dr. Fields: We have now come to the point where we need to direct our attention to the question of how some of these drugs are metabolized and try to relate what is known of the metabolism to what we are now learning about the influence on platelet function.

PART III

PHARMACOLOGY OF SALICYLATES

Moderator

Dr. William S. Fields

Chapter X

THE KINETIC DISPOSITION OF ASPIRIN IN HUMAN*

SIDNEY RIEGELMAN, PH.D.

Acetylsalicylic acid (ASA) is an extremely interesting compound which has been studied for a considerable number of years in man and animals. However, it has been possible only recently to accurately detect intact aspirin in the small quantities found in the body in the presence of large quantities of salicylic acid. Aspirin is rapidly absorbed from aqueous solutions and from solid dosage forms, with some degree of hydrolysis during the absorption phase and the first pass through the liver. It is then converted rapidly into salicylic acid in the blood, predominantly in the liver, although there is definitely hydrolysis of aspirin by other sites. These include the blood cells, plasma and kidney esterases. Approximately 30% to 50% of the orally administered doses are hydrolyzed before they reach the blood stream. The percent of hydrolyzed drug may vary to an amount larger than this, depending upon the dosage form used. Additional studies of this would be warranted in the future. The reason for the degree of hydrolysis during the first pass has been shown to be related to esterases located in the gut wall, plus the high clearance of the compound by the liver during the first pass.

Study of the data obtained from *in vitro* evaluation of the hydrolysis rate of the drug in whole blood or in plasma, as well as studies of the disappearance of the compound after administering an I.V. dose to the same humans, tentatively leads to the conclusion that as much as 25% of the hydrolysis may be due to reactions taking place in the blood (blood cells and plasma enzymes). It is my understanding that evidence has been obtained

---

from studies of ASA radio-tagged on the acetyl group, that hydrolysis results in a transesterification reaction with a significant uptake of radioactive acetyl groups by the blood platelets.

Studies of the blood levels of aspirin after I.V. administration at three-dose levels indicate that aspirin kinetics is unchanged. In other words, the compound follows dose independent kinetics. The resultant curves are biexponential in character, indicating some distribution into the tissues. The terminal half-life for the compound varies from 13 to 20 minutes in the tested subjects.

Figure 1 represents the data for aspirin and its resultant metabolite, salicylic acid, during the two-hour period after its oral administration as in aqueous solution. The curve is plotted on linear coordinate paper. It is noted in this individual that the blood levels peaked at approximately 22 μg in approximately 15 minutes and fell off rapidly. In 90 minutes to two hours, virtually all of the intact aspirin had disappeared from the blood. The rapid appearance of salicylic acid in the blood from the hydrolyzed aspirin is indicated by the dashed curve with the open triangles.

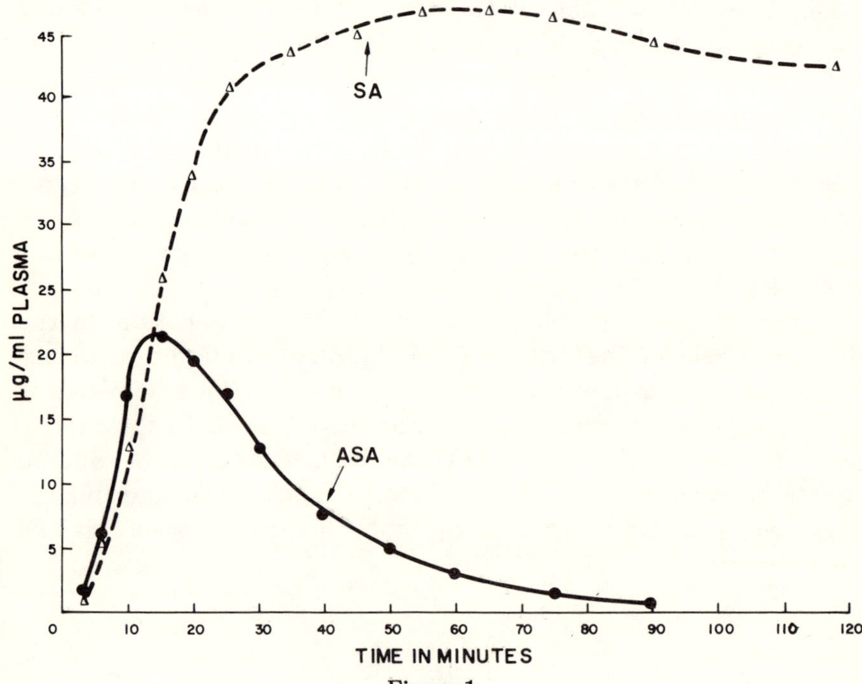

Figure 1.

The data is from a 650 mg dose. If larger doses of aspirin are given, a marked change is seen in the disappearance of salicylic acid from the blood. This will be discussed to some degree later.

Figure 2 represents the study of I.V. and oral solutions of aspirin in another test subject, both being administered at 650 mg.

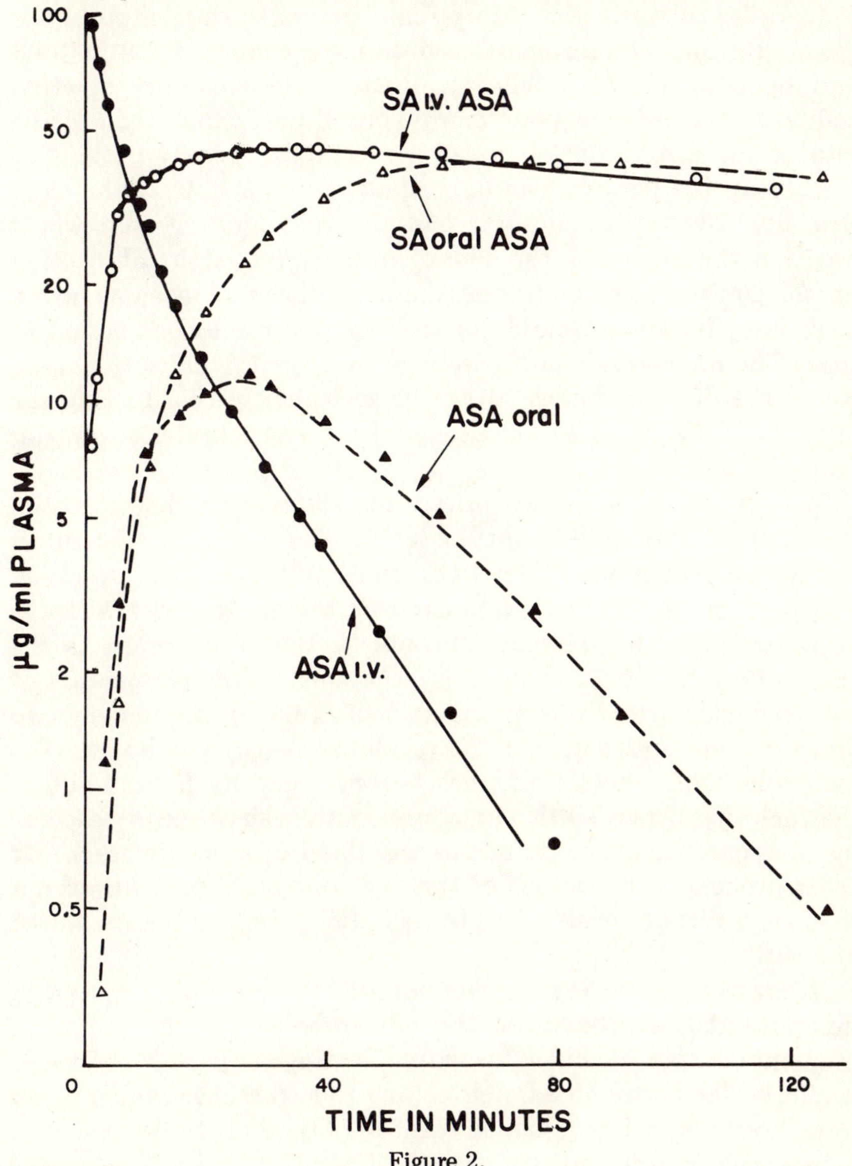

Figure 2.

It is to be noted that the curve indicated for the orally administered aqueous solution of aspirin does not exactly parallel that of the terminal phase of the curve. This is because absorption continues on a first order basis during at least the first 80 to 90 minutes.

In order to verify the absorption characteristics of aspirin, our research group administered the drug intravenously by an extract entrapped in an ethyl cellulose matrix. The solubility of ethyl cellulose is extremely poor in aqueous fluids, which reduces the rate of the dissolution of the aspirin crystals, thereby prolonging the absorption period. Aspirin is rapidly eliminated from the body (half-life 13 to 20 minutes) and the rate limiting step which controls the shape of the blood level curves is the absorption phase. Under these conditions, the drug does not reach as high a peak level but is detectable in the blood for a longer period of time. The data shown in Figure 8 is on a typical subject, administered the 650 mg dosage. It can be seen that in this instance the drug could be detected at 0.2 μg/ml for 264 minutes (over four hours).

It is important to review briefly the elimination characteristics of aspirin metabolite--salicylic acid. The latter compound is eliminated predominantly as its glycine conjugate, salicyluric acid. The percent of the dose eliminated by this route varies with the dose, as does the elimination rate of the compound. As the amount of the drug in the body accumulates, the elimination of salicylic acid varies from an original half-life of approximately two hours to an apparent half-life as long as twenty hours. The metabolism of salicylic acid has become capacity limited due to the fact that when sufficient concentrations have been reached, the enzymes are unable to metabolize the drug as an apparent first order process. It is because of this that one must be cautious not to exceed certain levels of aspirin administration in the treatment of arthritis.

It appears to me that application of the above information to the potential treatment of thromboembolism might require a frequent dosage regimen for administering aspirin. I believe it would be far better to administer one to two aspirin tablets every three hours or, if the sustained form were used, it would be logical to administer it logarithmic input. The blood samples obtained from this subject were analyzed for the apparent absorption characteristics by comparison of this blood data with that obtained previously from an I.V. dose of the drug. It was shown by this procedure that one could define the absorption characteristics of the compound quite precisely. This is shown in Figure 3 where the insert, upper right, indicates the percent remaining to be infused (absorbed). The line represents the theoretical input rate while the squares represent the experimental data.

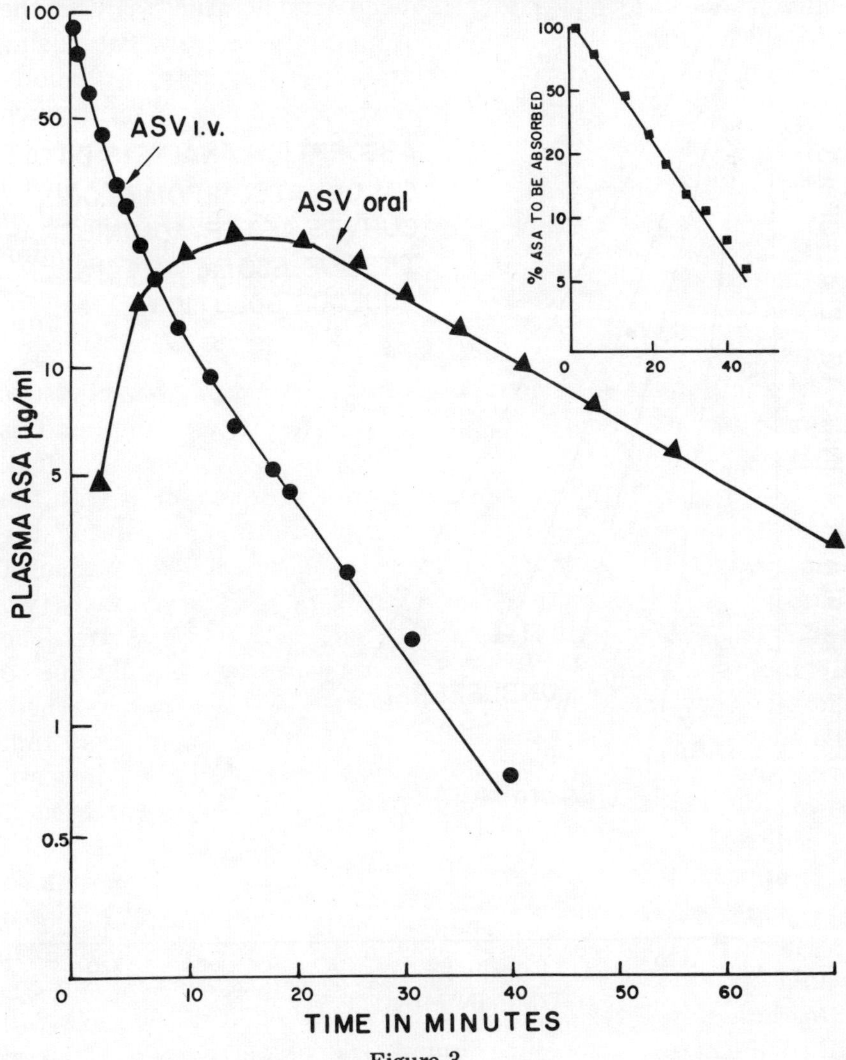

Figure 3.

Utilizing the same procedure, absorption of aspirin was followed in four subjects from a 650 mg aqueous solution of the drug. These are noted in Figure 4 as the percent remaining to be absorbed from aqueous solutions. It is seen that the absorption half-lives varied from approximately 4.5 to 22 minutes in the various subjects.

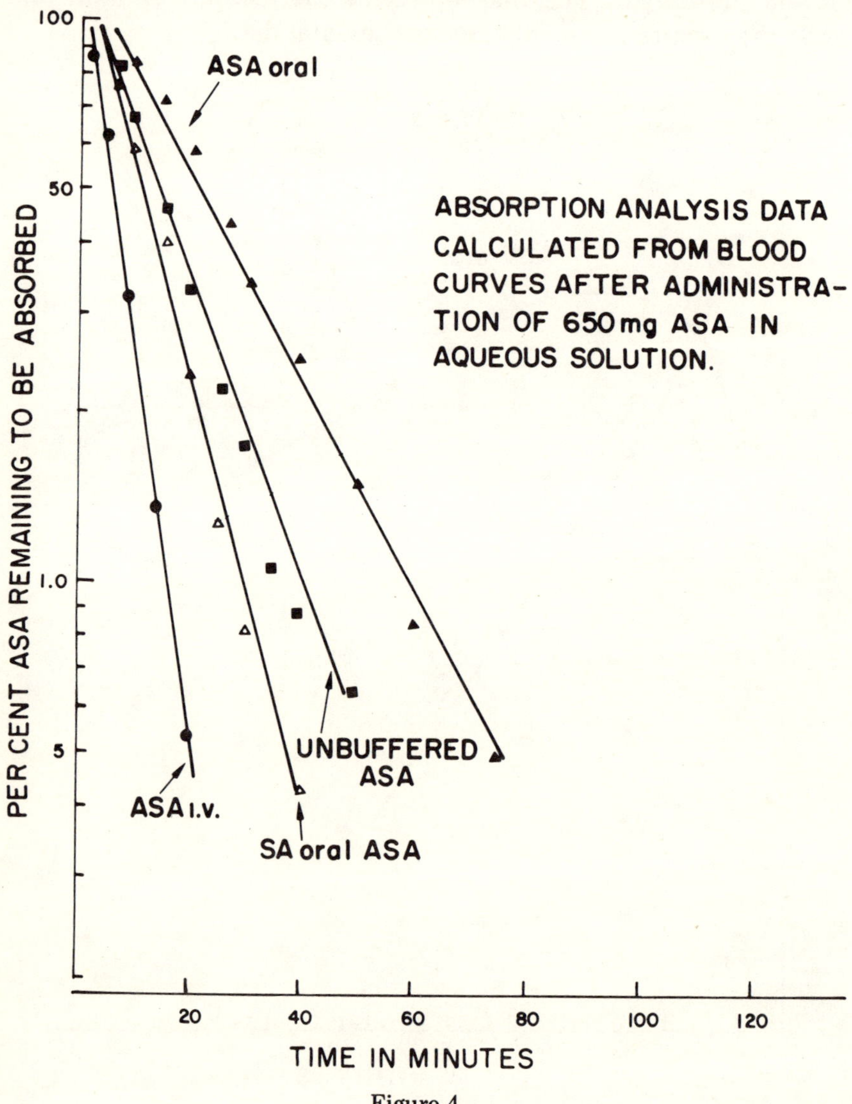

Figure 4

Absorption of aspirin from oral dosage varies remarkably from person to person. Figures 5-7 illustrate the aspirin blood levels after an I.V. dose administered as buffered and unbuffered aspirin. In some instances, the blood level during the first 20 minutes is markedly higher in buffered aspirin than it is in unbuffered aspirin. However, in our studies some subjects showed faster

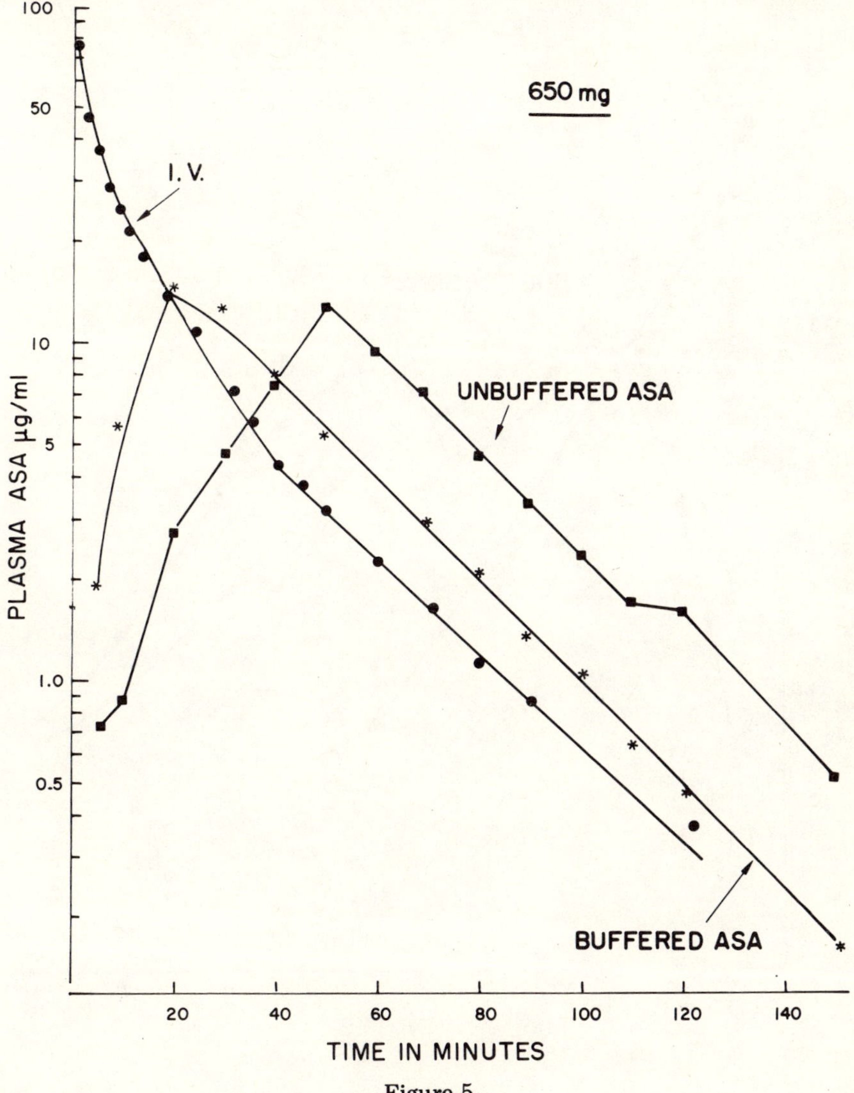

Figure 5

absorption from the unbuffered aspirin. The vast majority of the studies of aspirin tablets show the drug peaking at 10 to 20 minutes, and the peak value being sustained 10 to 12 μg/ml over a period of approximately 30 minutes, occasionally longer. The

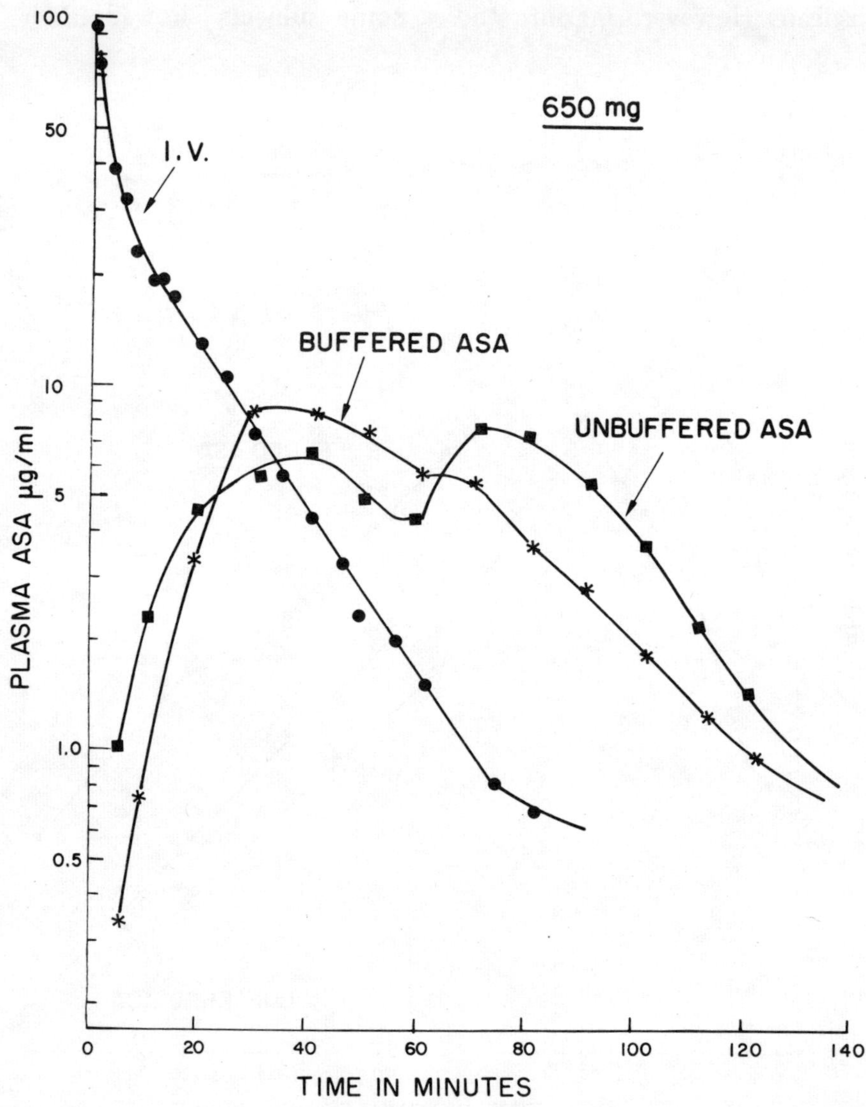

Figure 6

usual commercial aspirin products show minimum detectable blood levels of 0.2 μg/ml at approximately two hours.

Aspirin is, of course, available in a number of different commercial products in a sustained release form. One of these was tested in our laboratory, namely, Measurin. In this product, the release is every four hours. A continuum of intact aspirin could be

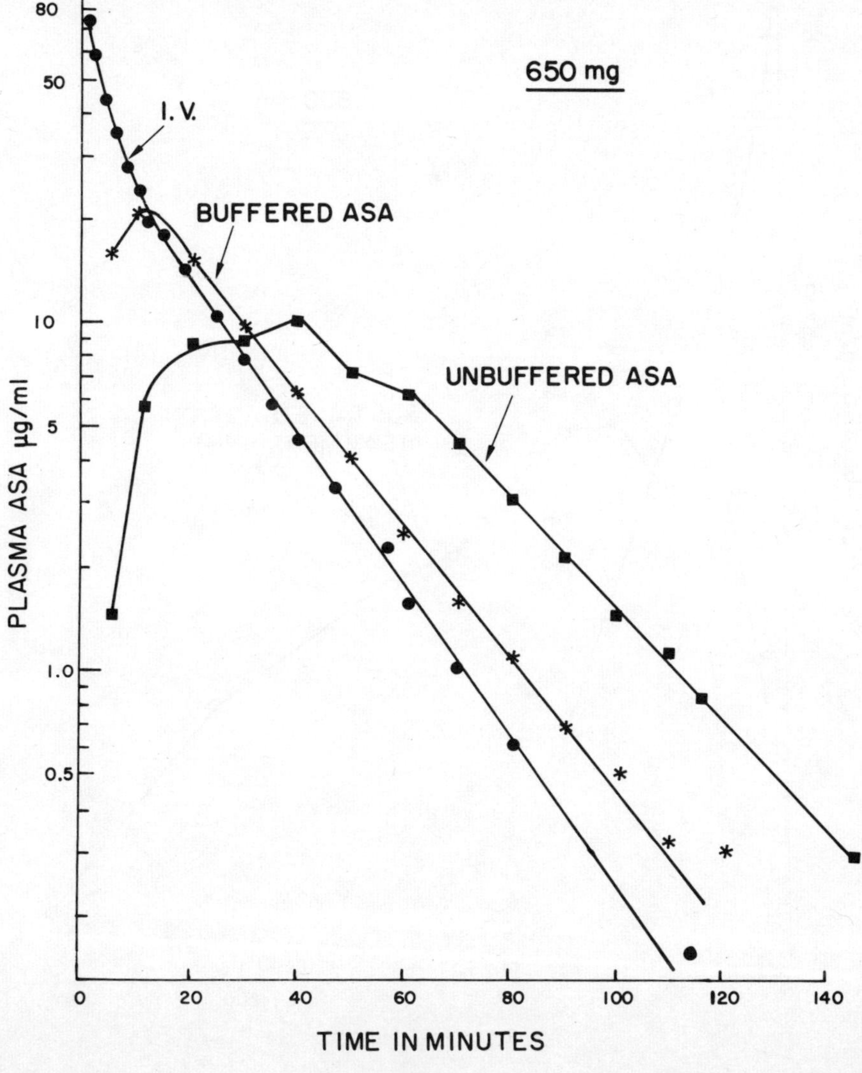

Figure 7

in the blood through much of the day with either regimen. Whether the levels are high enough for therapeutic activity will have to be judged by independent information not available to this author.

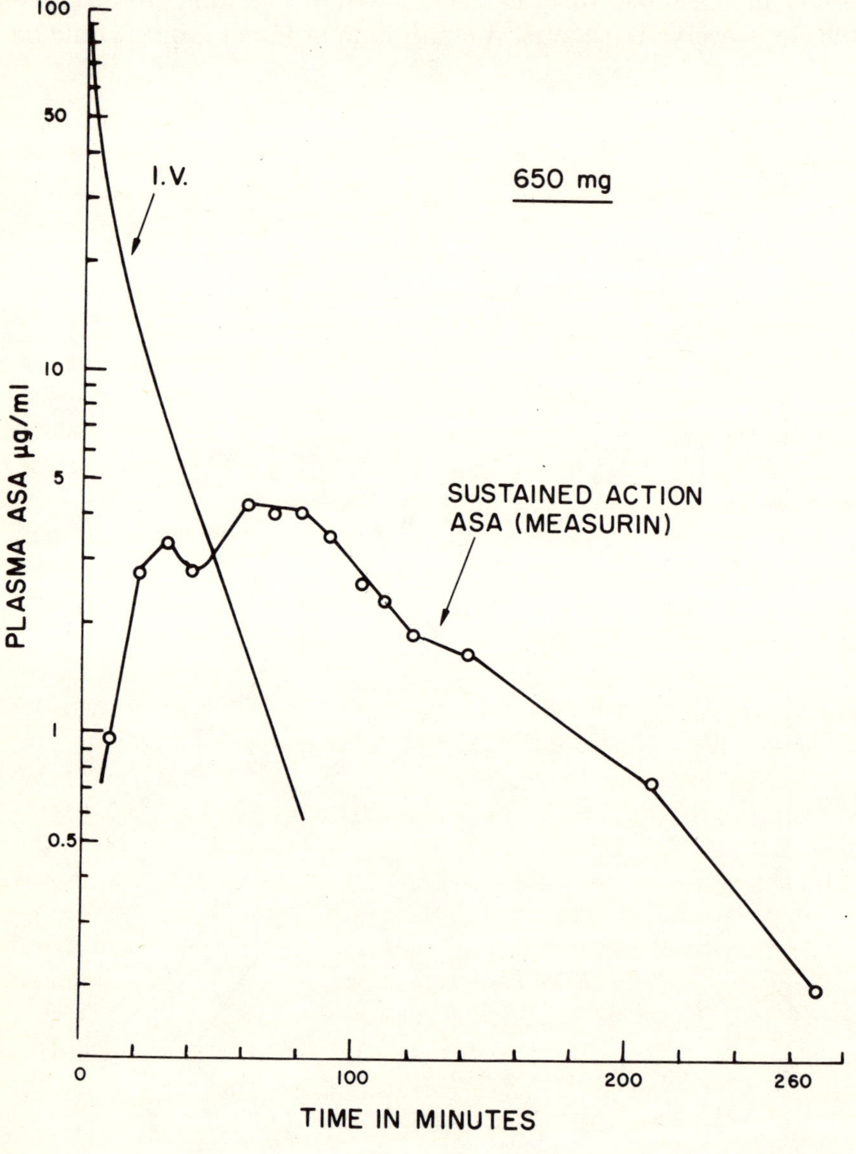

Figure 8

Chapter XI

METABOLISM OF SALICYLATES

EDWARD B. TRUITT, JR., PH.D.

I should begin with some apologies that are necessary to explain the presentation to follow. Dr. Fields caught me about two hours before I left for Washington for a three-day alcoholism conference--that was the subject of the research, not the activity of the participants. I barely had time to assemble some data, largely work that is several years old which was supported by the Bristol-Myers Company, one of the sponsors of this conference. I apologize, because I have not really been very active in salicylate research lately. I would like to draw heavily on Dr. Riegelman's comments, because he has been one of the forerunners in the study of the pharmaco-kinetics of salicylate drugs.

This position of the pharmacologist on the program, as you might recognize, is unusual. It is usually the reverse; that is, the pharmacologist is supposed to answer unasked questions first, and then the clinical questions come up and are unanswerable. But I think it is much nicer this way, where the clinical questions have been presented first and, hopefully, pharmacology can be appreciated a little more as being necessary for some answers.

One of the questions that is relevant today, and which has already been engaged, is: What is the molecular form of aspirin that is involved in this reaction of the platelets? What is the therapeutically active form of the drug that is affecting these ischemic episodes? Also, we need to ask: Is the action related to the rather prolonged salicylic acid levels that can result from therapeutic doses of aspirin, or is it related to the unhydrolyzed aspirin levels which last for a shorter period? Then, the other question which I suggested previously: Is the action related to some effect of the acetylated aspirin that outlasts, by a considerable length of time, the duration of the intact molecule in the bloodstream, i.e., a hit-and-run effect.

There are many clinical and pharmacological clues which rather strongly support the theory that at least some of the actions of aspirin or of salicylates are produced by the unhydrolyzed molecule. For example, it has already been pointed out that aspirin produces bleeding, perhaps more so than salicylic acid.

There are some experimental forms of erythema and irritation produced by chemical compounds in which aspirin is much more effective in inhibiting this phlogistic effect than the salicylate ion, i.e., hydrolyzed acetylsalicylate (1). There is another pharmacological test involving administration of irritants into the peritoneal cavity of mice. The animals go into a writhing type of motion that seems to be connected with the irritation, and aspirin is much more effective than sodium salicylate in this test, as well (2).

We often measure aspirin analgesia by a process of intra-arterial injection of a polypeptide, bradykinin, which produces in various organs a rather marked pain response. Aspirin is much more effective in blocking this peripheral action on pain receptors than is the hydrolyzed salicylate (3). Also using bradykinin, Collier has shown that the bronchoconstriction produced is much more antagonized by aspirin, about 30 times more so than by sodium salicylate (4).

Another difference that has been known--and mainly there is a sort of clinical feeling on this, rather than good scientific evidence--is that aspirin is a much better analgesic, especially for headache, than sodium salicylate (5). I understand that there have been two unpublished reports by Lasagna and Houde alluding to this fact. We also know that the duration of analgesia by aspirin probably parallels the short time period during which the unhydrolyzed aspirin remains in the blood, rather than the more prolonged salicylate levels.

These clues, I believe, lead to a consideration of some of the basic processes of aspirin in the body and of its metabolism. Unhydrolyzed aspirin, entering through the esophagus, is partially hydrolyzed in the stomach. Also, there is drug transport across the gastric membrane, without the necessity for stomach emptying, that can deliver into the circulation both the unhydrolyzed drug and the little bit of hydrolyzed drug that is formed there. The stomach is acidic, so there is usually not as rapid hydrolysis as there would be in an alkaline environment. As the pH of the stomach rises, emptying occurs; and there is another drug transport system across the intestinal membrane, in which some of the studies by Dr. Riegelman and others have demonstrated an enzyme system capable of producing hydrolysis. This is probably responsible for the transport of most aspirin to the blood. So there is considerable attrition of unhydrolyzed aspirin, due to aqueous hydrolysis and enzymatic hydrolysis, before the drug arrives in the bloodstream.

Distribution kinetics for the drug into the various tissue compartments must also be considered. Into the liver, there is a one-way process, resulting in metabolism and excretion. At this conference, we have been interested in the brain, of course, as it is affected by aspirin. There is a possibility that you might consider aspirin as a transport form of acetyl moieties to the brain, or of the intact drug to act neurally.

In studies we conducted several years ago for the Bristol-Myers Company and published in the Journal of Pharmaceutical Science, we showed that aspirin hydrolysis is extremely fast. It is, of course, hydrolyzed in solution, but in blood or plasma the hydrolysis rate is extremely accelerated by an enzymatic process, as was shown from some of Dr. Riegelman's data.

Acetylsalicylic acid (ASA), or unhydrolyzed aspirin levels rise rapidly, and continue high for only a short period. The levels of hydrolyzed salicylate rise as the unhydrolyzed fall. There are differential methods of measuring the two. Dr. Riegelman, I believe, used thin layer processes. We have used more wet chemistry methods that are perhaps a little less sensitive, but still capable of measuring the lower levels that exist during the first hour after administration. However, most of the free or unhydrolyzed aspirin is largely gone in about an hour.

After intravenous aspirin administration, the rapid rate of disappearance has two phases. There is an initial, very steep decline in the curve, where both distribution into tissues and hydrolysis is proceeding, and then a more linear phase, where the rate is principally that of hydrolysis. One can see by comparing the intravenous curve to that of the oral route that the latter produces more persistent levels of unhydrolyzed aspirin.

We have shown, as has Dr. Riegelman, that there is individual variability and wide variation in the overall level of aspirin remaining in the gut for absorption. There is ordinarily a linear rate of aspirin remaining to be absorbed. This is based on a sort of presumption, which was criticized recently by groups at Buffalo because it was not calculated by direct measurement of stomach contents. It was an indirect assumption derived from the plasma curves.

There have been comparative pharmacological studies to search for a test animal with an hydrolysis rate comparable to humans. Rats are perhaps a little faster, as far as aspirin hydrolysis is concerned, and this interestingly accounts for some of the difficulties which pharmacologists have encountered in using rats for certain analgesic studies. They were never able to show sufficiently good analgesia in rats when aspirin was compared with morphine. However, rabbits and cats have rates which are pretty close to humans. Some other animals that have also been used are a little too slow in aspirin hydrolysis to compare with the human. So, in considering animal studies, I think one has to be selective of the species.

We investigated a large number of laboratory volunteers for rate of hydrolysis. These showed variations of the rate. The test consisted of aspirin added to blood *in vitro,* and then the reaction was stopped at different intervals. The percentage of conversion was measured by increasing the optical density of the color reaction of free salicylate. It occurs quite rapidly, as observed in the *in vitro* data. When these rates are calculated as "K" values, it may be seen that there is a ten-fold range in the values. Some of the subjects under investigation absorbed salicylate very promptly, so that there was almost complete absorption in 20 minutes; while others were observed at 80 minutes with some unabsorbed drug remaining. There are a number of factors one can consider in this, particularly gastric emptying, mucous, the presence of food, and other impediments to absorption.

I think further study of the rates of absorption is indicated because the subjects to date were "normal" volunteers. Particular consideration should be given to a study of patients with rheumatoid arthritis who take large doses of aspirin. Studies of other pathologic conditions related to the rate of hydrolysis must be undertaken, as well.

The graphs presented by Dr. Riegelman show some of the complexities of considering the fate of aspirin in the body and the reactions that must be considered in setting up computer programs of the predictability of the drug and blood levels.

When one compares the absorption rates of buffered and unbuffered aspirin, it is obvious that there is prompt absorption in the buffered variety in contrast to the regular one. This is a real difference which we now believe to be related to the dissolution rate of aspirin in the stomach. The acceleration is rather significant and promotes slightly higher peak levels. Certainly, if the initial absorption rate and the peak height of the blood level are important, accelerated absorption through the use of buffers would be worthwhile considering in any therapeutic trial which one might wish to undertake.

Furthermore, when one considers the absorption of buffered vs. unbuffered aspirin, one sees on occasion a secondary peak that is most likely the result of gastric emptying. This event increases the total surface area, and thus increases the absorption rate, although initially the absorption rate was beginning to fall.

Other studies have been done with a product known as Measurin, which has been promoted as a sustained release form of acetylsalicylic acid. One must consider this claim very critically, however, in relation to the problem of absorption. If the delivery of the unhydrolyzed aspirin into the bloodstream is one's objective, then Measurin produces a prolonged, low level delivery of unhydrolyzed aspirin. This has been well demonstrated by Dr. Riegelman. However, it has also been shown that this is not necessarily true for higher doses. The result may be true for one or two tablets, but if one takes four tablets, the difference between the curves for the sustained-action product and the unmodified product disappears. There is a reason for this, in that the levels of salicylate are limited by metabolism and excretion mechanisms. Once these are saturated, there is no longer much difference in the total levels of salicylate between the two products. Measurin does, as I have suggested, have a limitation on its initial rate of delivery of high ASA levels.

There is one other aspect that neither Dr. Riegelman nor I have as yet discussed, which is important to this kinetic viewpoint of the aspirin problem. This concerns the binding of aspirin and salicylates to plasma proteins, which is an effective means of inactivating, temporarily and reversibly, the aspirin that is present. This problem has to be considered in patients who have marked variations in their total proteins and, in particular, the albumin fraction, which is the site of binding for most of the salicylate products.

Plasma binding, which will alter both the pharmacological action and the blood levels of aspirin, must be considered if we are going to be concerned with free aspirin, particularly the ability of free aspirin to hydrolyze and yield acetyl moieties.

You should be able now to recognize the complexities of aspirin delivery and the measurement of aspirin effect. This is obviously not a simple process. It has to be considered along with many other kinetic reactions, and the influence of one on the other as the process of metabolism proceeds.

Limitations of time make it necessary for me to omit a great deal of information concerning the further metabolism of aspirin, particularly to salicyluric acid, the glycine-coupled product of aspirin. I must also omit discussion of glucuronides that are formed, both the acetyl glucuronide and the phenolic glucuronide--two different products formed by glucuronide coupling.

There is another product known as gentisic acid which occurs with further hydrolyzation of the aspirin molecule, and this also needs to be considered in the overall metabolism.

Because of the apparent concern of the group attending this conference about the early absorption of aspirin and the levels of unhydrolyzed aspirin, I have tried to place emphasis on this phase.

REFERENCES

1. Adams, S.S., and Cobb, R.: In *Salicylates: An International Symposium.* Dixon, A.St.J., Martin, B.K., Smith, M.J.H., and Wood, P.H.N. (eds.). Boston, Mass., Little Brown & Co., 1963.
2. Siegmund, E.A., *et al.:* A method for evaluating both non-narcotic and narcotic analgesics. *Soc. Exp. Biol. &Med., 95*:729-731, 1957.
3. Lim, R.K.S., *et al.:* Site of action of narcotic and non-narcotic analgesics determined by blocking bradykinin-evoked visceral pain. *Arch. Int. Pharmacodyn., 152*:25-58, (Nov.) 1964.
4. Collier, H.O.J.: In *Salicylates: An International Symposium.* Dixon,

A.St.J., Martin, B.K., Smith, M.J.H., and Wood, P.H.N. (eds.). Boston, Mass., Little Brown & Co., 1963.

5. Leonards, J.R.: In *Proceedings of the Conference on Effects of Chronic Salicylate Administration.* Lamont-Haven, R.W., and Wagner, B.M. (eds.). Washington, D.C., USPHS Publ., 1966.

DISCUSSION OF CHAPTERS X AND XI

Dr. Fields: The preceding material should be very helpful. Certainly one of the things that we will find necessary is the resolution of the paradox concerning rapid hydrolysis and the prolonged effect on platelet function. I would hope that some of the other pharmacologists present would comment about this.

Dr. William Blackmore, Albany, N.Y.: Doctors Truitt and Riegelman certainly outlined the complexities of aspirin metabolism, and I would like to add a few comments. If a study were designed and set up to prove or disprove the role of aspirin in any one of several formulations, under conditions that we have been discussing, there are three or four points that I would suggest be kept in mind. They are based on several years of clinical experience with aspirin in various formulations.

One is that this would be a new use for aspirin, and the Food and Drug Administration would evaluate it in this respect. I think it will be necessary, therefore, to obtain blood level and urine samples. Although the FDA does not necessarily recognize that you can specifically correlate blood levels of acetysalicylic acid and salicylic acid with the onset, duration and degree of analgesia; nevertheless, I think they will want some type of bio-availability studies.

There are a tremendous number of methods of analysis available, and these many different methods are available because there is no one good method. If a study is set up, it is imperative that the best methodology for analysis be utilized. We conducted a double blind study a few years ago, using three different methods, with three independent laboratories, under strictly identical conditions. After the bloods were drawn, they were kept frozen for the same period of time so they would be run identically. It was amazing the great variability we obtained, and we ended up with two methods that have proven to be reproducible and very similar, and have adopted both methods. Therefore, I think that everyone is going to have to use one or two methods under identical conditions.

We also observed that if you freeze samples and then analyze for acetylsalicylic acid and salicylic acid, the salicylic acid levels over a period of time remain fairly constant, but after a two-week period you start detecting a decrease in acetylsalicylic acid levels. This effect would have to be considered since, if one laboratory ran analyses within ten days and another laboratory accumulates them because of time and facilities and runs them six months later, the salicylic acid may turn out to be satisfactory, but on the basis of our experience, the acetylsalicylic acid levels will be markedly different.

Another problem which I am sure everyone has encountered is the tremendous variability among individuals. We occasionally find an individual who develops a tremendous blood level of acetylsalicylic acid and salicylic acid with any type of aspirin formulation, buffered or plain.

Still another point to keep in mind in a study is standardization of the time of day when the samples are drawn. Diet can be a factor, and if the individual is taking an occasional drink of alcohol, this can also be a factor. We have found that some particular foods can play a role.

Dr. Fields: We are going to have to take many of these factors into consideration. When we come to consideration of experimental design, perhaps some of these questions can be discussed further and in greater detail.

Dr. Ben Marr Lanman, New York, N.Y.: I agree with Dr. Blackmore about the Food and Drug Administration. From a legal standpoint, you are going to have to file before you do any of these studies. We know that aspirin is used in larger doses for analgesia, but you are employing it for an entirely different purpose. According to the law, you will have to file for an I.N.D. (Investigator of New Drug) number, because aspirin is not recognized as safe and effective for this particular use.

Secondly, I do not know that your assay of levels during the treatment period is going to work out. Dr. Hass tells me he will be able to obtain blood samples from these people perhaps only every two or three weeks. I do not think you can get any useful data on the variation in levels of acetylsalicylic acid with that limited number of determinations. What do you think, Dr. Blackmore?

Dr. Blackmore: I agree with you; however, based on past experience, I cannot conceive of the Food and Drug Administration not requiring some bio-availability studies.

Dr. Lanman: It must be pointed out to them at the very beginning that one cannot do such studies as that, and should not be expected to because there are so many variables.

Dr. Blackmore: I agree with you one hundred percent, but I think you are going to be required to get some of these data, regardless of their significance.

Dr. Raymond Bauer, Detroit, Mich.: It seems that one of the better reasons for obtaining the levels would be to check the controls, i.e., to see that they are not taking aspirin. If we are going to use something as common as aspirin, we will have to check the controls rather carefully.

Dr. Fields: We may be getting a little off the subject under discussion, but I think that the experimental design must take into account the things that have been brought up here, such as the legal aspect, the bio-assay aspect, and certainly the epidemiological and biostatistical aspects. We will come back to these matters later.

Dr. Kantor: About this business of the blood levels, it is my understanding that two tablets three times a day would be more than sufficient aspirin for the effect desired. If you use aspirin in somewhat of an excess, I do not believe you are going to have to worry too much about the individual pharmacology of the drug.

Dr. Truitt: I believe it would be advisable to know whether these patients were fast or slow hydrolyzers of aspirin and whether they had rapid absorption or slow absorption of the drug, because it may be essential to the therapeutic effect that you are measuring. If it is, as assumed, a transacetylation process, it would require absorption of unhydrolyzed aspirin. It would be important, therefore, to know whether or not these people are absorbing the drug fast enough to produce effective levels of intact acetylsalicylate. This could be done in a preliminary test before the subjects are put on the longer study. Also, this would eliminate the need for obtaining long-term blood level data. You would categorize individuals, initially, as to their type of salicylate absorption.

Dr. Fields: There have been a number of studies mentioned here in which aspirin has been given to patients for this specific purpose. We would certainly not want to have it appear that people who have been working in this field have been doing so contrary to the requirements of the Food and Drug Administration. Therefore, before undertaking a controlled drug trial, we should certainly obtain proper advice about these matters.

Dr. Zucker: It seems you would be in an impossible bind if you wanted to check up on the patients. Would it, perhaps, be more to the point to test their platelet function and/or their urine? Even then, I do not know how you are going to check on them, because they may take their aspirin only for the two days before they come in to be checked.

Dr. Lanman: I think Dr. Kantor is right. The data shown earlier suggest that the amounts required to produce the desired effect are very low doses of aspirin. Even in the slow absorbers, they remained well within doses that he suggested, so I think two tablets a day would do it without much problem. Even if you gave them two tablets three times a day you would have no problem. You can establish this empirically, without having to draw blood samples from these people or having to go through very complicated analysis of urine or any other material. I believe the data already presented showed that very clearly.

Dr. Kantor: I just want to point out that I can speak as a rheumatologist, to whom six aspirin tablets a day for years is mere "chicken feed." We achieve that level in numerous patients without any difficulty whatsoever, so it would not be unreasonable to maintain a large population for a long period of time on this dose.

There is a question I would like to ask, however. Something that disturbed me about Dr. Weiss' presentation was the effect of epinephrine, which I gathered Dr. Zucker is not so sure about. Since we are looking, really, for both aggregation and adhesiveness, is there an effect here that we should consider? I think Dr. Truitt alluded to this in terms of vasoactive amines. Should we select another drug to take care of a second effect, or does this really exist as a problem?

Dr. Weiss: I am not sure I understand the question, Dr. Kantor.

Dr. Kantor: Is there an epinephrine effect which is not controlled by aspirin?

Dr. Weiss: As I indicated previously, the addition of epinephrine to platelet-rich plasma results in two waves of platelet aggregation. The first, and usually smaller wave is due to epinephrine itself; the second is the result of adenosine diphosphate (ADP) release from the platelets by epinephrine. The effect of aspirin is to inhibit platelet ADP release. Hence, only the second wave of epinephrine-induced aggregation is abolished by aspirin.

Dr. Kantor: Since epinephrine is obviously going to be circulating, would you think it worthwhile to control that feature?

Dr. Weiss: I think you are asking whether there may be other drugs which may be more effective than aspirin in inhibiting platelet function. Are there, for example, agents which may interfere with platelet adhesion, or abolish the first as well as the second wave of epinephrine-induced aggregation? There are agents with such properties, and I do not mean to infer that aspirin is necessarily the ideal agent.[1] For the kind of study we are proposing, however, we would like to use an agent which is safe, simple to administer, and whose side effects are well known. Aspirin would appear to be the drug which best fulfills these requirements at present.

Dr. Truitt: There is some data concerning interaction of aspirin with biogenic amines, particularly norepinephrine. The diagram (Fig. 1) illustrates the way in which I organize this interaction of epinephrine with platelet aggregation. If you consider the starting point of adenosine triphosphate (ATP), I think it has become apparent that the activity of ATP as a promoter of aggregation is largely by the action of NA+-K+-ATPase and the production of adenosine diphosphate (ADP). Then, by putting in epinephrine and serotonin (5-hydroxytryptamine) as a catalyzer of the ADP-promoted aggregation, you have a mechanism that is suggested to be inducing the added aggregation effect through further release of ADP.

Next, I should add that there is evidence that the alpha adrenergic blocking agents will block this aggregation effect, particularly by epinephrine.

Also, the conversion of ATP to cyclic adenosine monophosphate (AMP) by adenylcyclase has recently become of interest in

[1]Weiss, H.J.: Aspirin ingestion compared with bleeding disorders — Search for a useful platelet antiaggregant. *Blood, 35*:333-340, 1970.

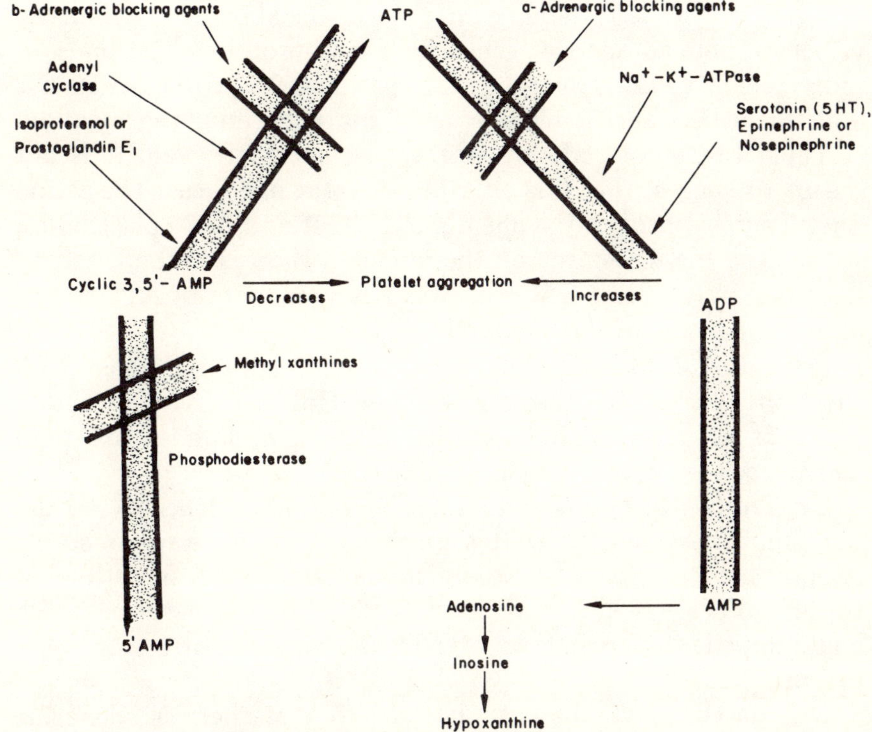

Figure 1. Hypothetical diagram of mechanisms for the action of adrenergic agonists and antagonists on platelet aggregation.

this area of platelet aggregation. This is because it has been shown that aggregation is inhibited by the action of cyclic AMP or dibutyryl cyclic AMP (which is really a more lipid-soluble form of cyclic AMP for interacting with receptors), and other ways of promoting the action of the cyclic AMP. The action is blocked by beta adrenergic blocking agents.

The system also interacts in another interesting way. Further metabolism of cyclic AMP produces 5^1-AMP through the action of phosphodiesterase, and this enzyme is inhibited by the methylxanthines, which also inhibit clotting. This, caffeine or theophylline products, by blocking the destruction of cyclic AMP, also seems to promote inhibition of aggregation.

It has been further theorized that the metabolism of ADP leads to adenosine and further to inosine and hypoxanthine, and that the action of persantine (dipyridamole) may be through interference with the breakdown of ATP to ADP.

Again on the left, the diagram gives us the ability to explain the effects of beta adrenergic agents, such as isoproterenol (isuprel) or, more recently, the prostaglandins, particularly prostaglandin E_1, which is a beta adrenergic-like agent and also inhibits aggregation.

Thus, the whole scheme works out amazingly well. It is not meant to suggest that this all takes place at one locus. The action on ATPase is probably a membrane effect and takes place either within the membrane or on the outside, whereas Sutherland and his group have shown that cyclic AMP is a mediator of ATP effects on the inner side of the membrane.

Dr. Aaron J. Marcus, New York, N.Y.: There is a problem with the right side of the diagram, because Holmsen has shown that platelets have a readily available adenosine diphosphate pool which does not come from adenosine triphosphate.

Dr. Truitt: That portion does not have good evidence to rest on, but some have suggested this mechanism as the way adenosine triphosphate works. Also, there are a number of inhibitors of Na^+-K^+-ATPase which will seem to fit this scheme also, which could impede the breakdown of ATP as a means of affecting aggregation.

Dr. Marcus: But Holmsen has shown that there is adenosine diphosphate that does come out during aggregation.

Dr. Truitt: Does this mean it was already there?

Dr. Marcus: It is not from adenosine triphosphate.

Dr. Truitt: Does he mean it is already there and available for release, or that at least it is not produced in the process?

Dr. Marcus: Right. There are two separate pools of adenosine triphosphate.

Dr. Truitt: Certainly the rapidity of adenosine diphosphate appearance would suggest that there is some already there, but its further production would be from adenosine triphosphate.

Dr. Fields: It is obvious from this discussion that there are still gaps in our understanding of these mechanisms. If we decide to undertake a controlled clinical trial, it will have to be based on our present knowledge. Concepts of normal and pathophysiologic mechanisms will change. As we learn more about them, we must be sufficiently adaptable to be able to utilize to the fullest advantage possible all new information as it becomes available.

PART IV

CONTROLLED CLINICAL TRIALS

Moderator

Reuel A. Stallones, M.D., M.P.H.

Chapter XII

EXPERIMENTAL DESIGN: A PANEL DISCUSSION

Panelists: DR. MARK DYKEN, DR. RALPH FRANKOWSKI, DR. WILLIAM S. FIELDS, and DR. CLARK H. MILLIKAN

Dr. Reuel A. Stallones, Houston, Tex.: This has been a very edifying experience for me. Before I came here, I had the idea that platelet "stickiness" was something that made you go to another restaurant.

I would not pretend in any group, much less this one, to be much of a medical historian, but controlled clinical trials are really a remarkable development of the last few years. Nearly all of this has developed since World War II, and during this time we have accumulated an enormous amount of experience.

The trial that is of most interest historically to epidemilogists is the polio vaccine field trial of 1954. This illustrated a number of very important considerations, one being that people would, indeed, voluntarily enter a study in which they knew that they--or in this case, their children--might or might not receive an agent which was presumed to be effective against a disease which had a massive emotional impact.

The various designs which have been used in this kind of undertaking are well known. There are a variety of them, but they are all based on a very simple precept: Concern with the relation between two events--something that is done to a person, and something which is observed at some time thereafter.

The rigidity of an experimental design is to attempt to assure that the second occurrence is reasonably attributable to the first, and that it is not reasonably attributable to something else. This, of course, leads to all kinds of ramifications with respect to the design, and to concern with biases that might disrupt such a study. The most common ones, I suppose, are (a) selection bias (how the people who are in the treated and untreated or variously treated groups relate to each other, how they compare with each other); (b) observer bias (what the experimenter contributes to the study which should not be there); and (c) the subject bias (which has also been called the "placebo effect").

The simplest answer to selection bias is random allocation of subjects to treated and untreated, or to various treatment groups. The ordinary answer to observer bias is that the study should be blind, and the ordinary answer to subject bias is that the study should be double blind.

One of Robert Heinlein's more interesting tales was about an aviator who crashed in a closed valley and discovered he was in the midst of a community where everyone was blind. Immediately, it occurred to him that a bit of folk wisdom should apply, that is, in the land of the blind, the one-eyed is king. Since he was doubly sighted, he thought that he would surely assume leadership in this community. Well, the story has an unhappy ending. Because of his evident visual hallucinations, the people who lived in this community were very much concerned about his mental health. Eventually, their scientists had him strapped down to a table and were prepared to enucleate the tumors that appeared on the front of his head which were obviously pressing on his brain and causing his difficulties. I believe there is a lesson in there for a double-blind study.

If a group differs, it must differ from something else, and the question is: From what does it differ? This leads us to a concern with expectation. What is the expected frequency of an event in the study population? How might one derive an expected value? Many people have a strong belief that an event should happen so many times, and if something differs from this strong belief, then it differs from expectation. Unfortunately, a strong belief is not easily quantifiable, and some people would choose, therefore, to develop an expectation based on their prior experience. If in 20 years of practice, a person has become accustomed to a certain frequency, he may believe that that constitutes a basis for a computable expectation of events. However, a more rigid and more solid expectation is based on an untreated control group.

This brings up the ethical issue of withholding treatment, which must be discussed in planning studies of this kind.

One thing which also came up during the discussions, and which I am sure will need further discussion here, is the effect of dilution. This is the effect on the study of people who are supposed to be taking a drug but who do not take it, and people who are not supposed to be taking a drug but who do take it. From an epidemiologic point of view, this is one of the more favorable kinds of biases that can occur, because it is not likely to produce spurious correlation between things, but rather to diminish a true correlation.

We have assembled a distinguished panel, and I will ask each of the panel members, in turn, if they would like to comment on some of the special problems in design that they see as affecting the proposal under consideration.

Dr. Dyken: We are gathered here today to discuss a cooperative study using aspirin in cerebrovascular disease. Several things have bothered me about this proposed study. First, aspirin is a drug that any idiot can buy in any quantity he chooses and take for whatever condition he chooses. There has been a great deal of experience using aspirin in a variety of conditions. Other than in high doses and with small children, there has been no serious trouble. Therefore, it would seem to be unrealistic to deny the use of aspirin in the low doses proposed for this study.

Second, can this study be done by one individual group or by several individual groups separately? I do not think there is a doubt in the minds of any of us who have participated in cooperative studies that the design is much cleaner if the study can be satisfactorily done with one group of investigators. A multiplicity of investigators provide data that, perforce, has to be different. Nevertheless, cooperative studies do have many advantages and sometimes are the only way to arrive at answers to your questions.

Finally, from past personal experience in cooperative studies, I would make a plea that the design be kept as simple as possible. One of the major difficulties in such studies is that frequently each of the individual investigators wants to learn something new or different, and the design becomes unwieldy. The simpler the hypothesis can be made, the more likely the study is to come up with definite answers. For instance, there are certain patients on whom this treatment should not be performed.

Dr. Millikan: Who are they?

Dr. Dyken: One could dilute the group of subjects by considering cerebrovascular disease. *in toto,* so that it would take thousands upon thousands of patients to come up with the results.

Dr. Millikan: Which ones should not get the treatment?

Dr. Dyken: If I were to design this study, I would think that it would have to be limited to patients who have a definable transient cerebral ischemic attack which fulfilled as many objective criteria as the investigators could agree upon. I would not include an individual with an established infarction. I would use as an end point either death or, as defined by all members, an irreversible dysfunction of the nervous system probably due to infarction.

These are just a few of the thoughts that have gone through my mind.

Dr. Ralph Frankowski, Houston, Tex.: I think that any comment which I might make at this time about the design would be a bit premature. As I have listened, I have heard suggestions for five or six or possibly more different types of trials. Possibly the only way that I can be of assistance to the group, if at all, is to suggest a reasonable manner in which to proceed so as to insure that adequate data will be collected once the objectives and criteria for the study have been developed. Furthermore, I would want to be sure that once the data are in, we could make an inference or judgment about them.

I would like to re-emphasize Dr. Stallones' point about the fundamental criteria that are developed for controlled trials. Very briefly, they are the elements of randomization, replication and controls. We have had controls of several sorts mentioned, including two or three types of current drugs, and even a suggestion of reconstructive surgery as an alternative mode of treatment.

First, we must reach a precise definition of both the population in which we are interested and the problem involved. We must also have a precisely defined response, whether it be platelet inhibition, or the recurrence or non-recurrence of transient or non-transient cerebral events. In the discussions about aspirin, several persons mentioned that there are going to be dosage problems. We are going to have to determine whether the medication will be administered orally or parenterally, and whether there are additional problems about absorption which will require solution. Until decisions of this nature have been made by the prospective investigators, I feel that I can be of only limited assistance.

There are other technical problems in addition to the problems already mentioned by Dr. Stallones. Later on, when a group of investigators discuss the detailed plan for a study, I will be pleased to make available to them a ten-page document of "Guidelines for Cooperative Trials," which I have in my files and which they may find helpful. It contains a series of "do's" and "don'ts" gathered from experience in the field. I would, therefore, suggest that when the objective of the study and the basic criteria for the collection of data are evolved, this might be matched with currently accepted guidelines for a controlled trial.

Dr. Fields: We are concerned with the proposition of giving a drug to a large population and trying to determine, in a prospective way, whether it is possible to prevent a stroke. This is what Dr. Tonks has done in an uncontrolled fashion in England, and he has come up with what appears to be a rather dramatic set of figures.

As far as defining population is concerned, I think Dr. Millikan brought out a question which will be crucial: Who should be in and who should be out? It appears from the material presented that the patient who is the most logical candidate for consideration is the one who is already symptomatic with cerebrovascular disease in the form of transient cerebral ischemic attacks. One facet of this problem is arriving at a concensus decision about what constitutes a transient cerebral ischemic attack.

Double blind studies of pharmacological agents are familiar to everyone attending this conference, but we must decide before undertaking an experimental trial what we mean by "double blind" and how rigidly we intend to adhere to our definition. Are we going to use two agents, which are identical in appearance but one of which is an active preparation and the other a placebo? Personally, from an ethical or moral standpoint, I cannot conceive of a "no-treat" group if we are to deal with symptomatic patients. Further, are we going to compare medical and surgical modes of therapy and, if so, will the same drugs be given to both the surgically and the non-surgically treated subjects.

In the controlled surgical trial, which is drawing to a close and in which we are now engaged in follow-up, it was decided at the outset that both the surgically and non-surgically treated groups would receive "the best available medical treatment." It was obvious that this would vary to some extent from one to the other of the participating institutions, often depending upon what was then in vogue. It was our hope, however, that any bias created by lack of a rigid definition of medical therapy would be offset by the random allocation of subjects to the two groups.

One of the principal criticisms of clinical therapeutic trials which have been done in the past on cerebrovascular patients has been that the anatomical lesion was not clearly defined. In the past decade, techniques have been developed to the point where the vascular lesion can be reasonably well defined in almost all cases by adequate arteriographic study. It is perfectly clear that the only reason for doing arteriograms will be to identify anatomically a specific lesion or lesions in order to proceed to the next logical step, namely, selection of specific therapy.

As Dr. Kricheff pointed out very carefully in his presentation, judicious employment of arteriography will enable us to select from a large population of persons symptomatic with cerebrovascular disease, those individuals who fit certain predetermined criteria. It was evident that the two surgeons whose presentations followed his were also in agreement on this point.

Another difficulty which is inherent in cooperative clinical trials is a tendency for the prospective participants to overestimate the number of subjects available. They state that they see a large number of patients who will meet the specified criteria, yet, when the moment of truth arrives, there are frequently not as many patients as the investigators originally thought they could include.

As director of a data registry, I can speak from experience about the problem of maintaining motivation and enthusiasm among a diverse group of investigators. Unfortunately, there is a long time between the in-put of information and the retrieval, analysis and out-put. This creates tremendous anxiety on the part of some persons in the individual institutions, particularly when they are under considerable pressure from their colleagues for answers to important questions. Unfortunately, these answers are not likely to be forthcoming until a sufficient period of time has elapsed and a large enough sample of subjects has been accumulated. Answers obtained too quickly, and under pressure, are likely to be inaccurate or misleading.

Participants in a cooperative study must be prepared to stick with it for the length of time which has been agreed upon at the outset, unless it becomes obvious at an early date that one or the other method of therapy is much better or much worse. Under either of these circumstances, it would not be ethical to continue. In other words, one must build into the design a clear understanding that when or if statistical significance is reached in a defined group of subjects in whom a particular form of therapy is obviously worse than another form of therapy, then it is no longer ethical or moral to continue to randomly allocate subjects to that group, and one must withdraw them from the trial.

These are just some of the problems that one needs to keep in mind in the development of this kind of undertaking.

Dr. Millikan: What is the question that is being asked?

Dr. Fields: The question that is being asked is whether there would be a reduction in transient cerebral ischemic episodes in the carotid territory, and subsequent infarction, by utilizing aspirin as a means of interfering with intra-arterial clotting. The choice of other methods of treatment with which it would be compared is a matter for further consideration.

Dr. Millikan: Traditionally, we refer to transient cerebral ischemic attacks as being in the carotid territory or in the vertebral basilar territory. There has been considerable confusion about these phrases. When originally designed, they had to do only with the clinical implication of the region of brain involved in the transient ischemic process. They did not, or were not intended to imply the site or sites of the arterial lesions which might or might not be defined if arteriography were performed. This is a very important issue since one frequently hears, at national meetings, that the diagnosis of transient cerebral ischemic attacks is made by arteriography. It should be obvious to all of you that the diagnosis of a transient cerebral ischemic attack cannot possibly be made with an arteriogram.

The diagnosis is made almost always on the basis of the history, except for those unusual circumstances where the physician may be present during the occurrence of such an attack. The morphology of the arterial system can be depicted quite precisely by the excellent arteriographic techniques available today; and, as several of you in this room have stated, it is possible for the arteriogram to be normal in a patient with classical transient cerebral ischemic attacks. Issues such as this are of great importance to you as you come to grips with the problem of defining transient cerebral ischemic attacks in your protocol.

Here is a caution: If you look at the literature that has developed on the natural history of transient ischemic attacks, you see some very interesting phenomena. Most of you are aware of the paper that John Marshall wrote a number of years ago, called "The Natural History of Transient Cerebral Ischemic Attacks." You are aware that he described three groups: I, II, and III. In Group II, there were 61 patients who presented with only transient cerebral ischemic attacks; their neurologic examinations were normal. Group I patients presented with a clinical picture of a previous cerebral infarction and, by history, had suffered transient cerebral ischemic attacks. If you read that paper, you found that all the discussion in the paper is about Group I. As you follow Group II, with 61 patients, for 47.5 months average, only one patient developed cerebral infarction. One, therefore, becomes very much interested in the definition of transient ischemic attacks in Group II. You cannot find the definition in the paper and you are left with a large percentage of patients having "dizziness and unsteadiness." Suddenly, he is talking about another group of patients. Certainly Group II did not consist of patients with transient cerebral ischemic attacks.

If you bring into the protocol for a future study such non-specific complaint phenomena as dizziness and unsteadiness, you will introduce a lack of specificity which will make your ultimate findings meaningless. You might decide that you want to study dizziness and unsteadiness as an isolated combination of complaints; and you might have 200 such people taking aspirin and 200 not. You might discover that aspirin was marvelous for dizziness and unsteadiness. It will not be realistic to think of such a category as representing the traditional transient cerebral ischemic attack patients.

If you get into the study of aspirin, define the terms precisely, ask a simple straightforward question, and keep laboratory involvement and all ancillary phenomena to a minimum. One question that will plague you is how to accurately establish that one category of patients being studied take the aspirin, and that the other category do not take it. You may find the latter task impossible.

You must make decisions concerning the inclusion or exclusion of reconstructive vascular surgery as the treatment. This will be a difficult matter, as there are now many individuals who believe it would be unethical to withhold surgery when a patient with transient cerebral ischemic attacks has both ulceration and stenosis due to atherosclerosis.

If you attempt to study the therapeutic effectiveness of aspirin on sub-divisions of patients, based on whether such sub-divisions have one or more characteristics of the stroke-prone profile, you will amost hopelessly complicate the investigation. If the sub-groups are to be set up on the basis of the presence or absence of obesity, hypertension, diabetes, cardiac disease, changes in the lipid profile, an abnormality of the electocardiogram, hyperuricemia, polycythemia, or abnormal thyroid metabolism, you will not be able to accomplish your task in a reasonable period of time.

Stay with your two original questions: (1) Does the chronic ingestion of aspirin produce a reduction in the number of transient cerebral ischemic attacks, and (2) does the chronic ingestion of aspirin decrease the risk of cerebral infarction associated with transient ischemic attacks.

Dr. Stallones: May we have general discussion from the floor?

Dr. Bauer: One of the first thoughts that comes to my mind, after listening to the discussion thus far, is the tendency to become "brainwashed" that all transient cerebral ischemic attacks are caused by emboli. They can be caused by emboli, but we do not want to fall into the trap of saying that they are all caused by emboli and forget about the other causes. So, right away, we have to make some decision in the proposed study as to which transient cerebral ischemic attacks we are going to include. If we include them all, then some further classification as to etiology is necessary. If we are using aspirin as treatment to prevent platelet aggregation, we have to do our best to compare only the patients who we think are clinically affected by platelet aggregation and resultant emboli.

Once patients are considered as eligible for the study, we will have to divide them into those eligible for surgical treatment and those not eligible for surgical treatment. It is possible that you are going to have two divisions of randomization, i.e., surgical and non-surgical patients, each group randomized into aspirin and no-aspirin medical treatment.

The non-surgical patients would include those with intracranial lesions. The patient who is non-operable could be randomized for aspirin vs. placebo, or whatever drug you decide to use as a control.

I personally feel that if you are going to make intelligent observations about the effects of aspirin, you are also going to need arteriography on at least the major portion of the patients.

The transient cerebral ischemic attack, by the present definition, is an event which is completely cleared within twenty-four hours. Maybe we will have to extend the time limit to include patients who have a complete clearing within a reasonable period of time--two days, four days, or even seven days.

Now, what about the patients whose transient cerebral ischemic attacks can be treated in some other way? What about the patient who comes in with undiagnosed diabetes? You treat the diabetes. Now, is he better because you treated the diabetes? Should you put him in the aspirin study? What about untreated hypertension? Are you going to treat the hypertension and give him aspirin or placebo and consider him in the study? What about the patient with cardiac arrhythmia? Are you going to put a cardio-monitor on and discover he is having transient ischemic attacks because of prolonged asystole, put him on a drug to improve his cardiac rhythm, and still put him in the study?

These are the types of questions we have to be considering now, rather than one year from now when we have 50 patients, or three years from now when we have 200 patients and wish we had "cleaned up" the design.

Dr. Richard Janeway, Winston-Salem, N.C.: Many of the things I had planned to say have already been said. Dr. Stallones has stated on other occasions that one must randomize; and indeed, in addition to random allocation, one must stratify; and then one must randomize within strata. If one does not, one gets into trouble. Once having randomized, and then randomized within strata, one must never look back, because it cannot do anything but make him unhappy.

Given the fact that you can define transient cerebral ischemic attacks--and I think that many of us here would use the same definition--and given the fact that aspirin quite clearly has an effect on platelet aggregation, you then come down, unfortunately, to trying to test two things. You are trying to abstract a pathophysiologic mechanism, the frequency of which you do not know in the population with which you are dealing. The situation becomes complicated.

If you are to answer a question, the easiest one is that which has only one variable, and all others can be eliminated. It seems to me that if one is testing a hypothesis of drug use and at the same time one is testing the validity and frequency of a pathophysiologic mechanism, there will be trouble arriving at an answer that is not inherently circular.

Dr. Holt McDowell, Birmingham, Ala.: From the surgeon's point of view, participation in this study will present some problems related to randomization that have been encountered and satisfactorily resolved in the previously mentioned Joint Study of Extracranial Arterial Occlusion. In this previous study, I was reluctant to randomize patients who had a 90% or greater area of stenosis. In other words, I cannot morally justify randomizing the hairline stenosis. The majority of the patients who will be studied arteriographically will be patients who I believe can be helped by some method of therapy. I, personally, would have wider indications for surgical intervention than others at this meeting; however, I believe that I would be flexible in most areas, except the aforementioned high grade stenosis.

In regard to the question raised as to the definition of a transient cerebral ischemic attack, I frequently see patients whose neurologic symptomatology is solely dizziness. It is very difficult for me to accurately determine exactly what is a "dizzy spell." The only patients that I feel confident have definitely experienced a transient cerebral ischemic attack are those who have experienced a definite sensory or motor deficit that was transient. I believe that a patient's history in regard to sensory and motor deficits is fairly reliable.

With reference to Dr. Millikan's remarks regarding hyperuricemia and all the other metabolic abnormalities that are encountered in patients such as those under discussion, I would think that it would be wise to eliminate them from the study. For example, if a patient is found to have myxedema during his evaluation, then this patient should not be in the study. To state it another way, I believe that we should have a few basic tests to eliminate patients whose symptoms are suggestive of transient cerebral ischemia but which are actually on the basis of diabetes, myxedema, etc.

Dr. Stallones: For most persons on whom you wish to operate, would you be prepared to randomly allocate them to aspirin and no aspirin, before and after operation?

Dr. McDowell: I would be willing to randomize all operative patients in regard to aspirin or no aspirin.

Dr. Stallones: It seems to me there was material earlier on preoperative aspirin as priming for persons subjected to endarterectomy.

Dr. McDowell: This morning Dr. Fields mentioned recovery room funduscopic visualization of embolic particles. I think that it would be of interest if one of our ophthalmology or neurology colleagues would observe every patient following carotid endarterectomy to see if there is any difference in the number of retinal embolic particles observed between an aspirin-treated group as opposed to a non-aspirin treated group. I would be willing to administer aspirin pre-operatively as well as post-operatively on a randomized basis on those patients subjected to surgery.

Dr. Hass: I would like to look through the other end of the telescope for a minute. Most of us who have worked in the cooperative extracranial arterial occlusion study are agreed that a patient who has a transient cerebral ischemic attack and a single carotid ulcerative lesion in the appropriate vascular territory makes a very good candidate for surgery, in experienced surgical hands. However, this feeling varies. One of the virtues of a cooperative study is that all participants do not feel the same way.

Some physicians at some institutions still feel that surgery should not be used in patients with transient cerebral ischemic episodes, except in patients who have ulcerative lesions or thrombus hanging in the vessel, such as Dr. Kricheff showed us. At my own institution, I am one of the few "pro-surgical" neurologists. The rest of them would prefer to administer medical therapy, often including anticoagulants. There are still varied opinions about surgery, and the situation is not at all clear-cut.

I envision a larger study which is not merely restricted to transient cerebral ischemic attacks, a study where the definition of stroke categories is very accurate, and where motor deficit, or aphasia, or other specific symptoms of cerebral dysfunction are the basis for the definition of the clinical categories. It will include transient cerebral ischemic attacks, with and without complete recovery, and even since this is a non-surgical program, patients who have had a completed stroke.

I envision, therefore, a three-tiered study. On one tier, a patient who presents at one of the many cooperating institutions will be well defined, angiographically and clinically. A certain number of this group, depending upon that institution's view of surgery, will be operated; and the other group will be randomized for medical therapy. Depending upon one's ethical feelings, they would be randomized for aspirin versus placebo, or aspirin versus sulfinpyrazone. I, myself, would have a very difficult time, knowing what I know now, randomizing aspirin against placebo. If I had a transient cerebral ischemic attack, I would like to have some aspirin or some sulfinpyrazone, in view of the present, albeit only suggestive, data. Where there were no concurrent controls, we would be forced to do retrospective analyses of untreated patients in previous carefully controlled studies as comparison groups, which introduces one of Dr. Stallones' suggested biases.

A second tier in this study would be similar to the study I described for dipyridamole in England. In many institutions, referring physicians and many full-time physicians still do not want their patients who have clear-cut transient or persistent stroke syndromes to be subjected to angiography. We do not all agree on indications for angiography, and this is probably a good thing. In this second tier, we might lack the angiography, but we would certainly have more patients. These, then, could be randomized according to a protocol we would develop for, shall we say, aspirin versus sulfinpyrazone or aspirin versus placebo.

A third, even more general, tier could be something which has been envisioned by one of the members of my own school. This would involve a group of elderly patients in a restricted environment who could be carefully observed. One half of this group of patients would receive aspirin, and one half placebo. This elderly population would not necessarily be characterized by previous cerebrovascular disease. In the randomization process we would probably, if we had sufficient numbers, have rather similar population groups. In this population, the end point of the study would again be the same as in the other tiers: Significant reduction of the incidence of transient cerebral ischemic attacks, as carefully defined, or stroke, through employment of drug therapy during the study period.

So, I offer the other end of the telescope to try to get this effort going on as many levels as possible.

Dr. Stallones: Dr. Ehrenfeld

Dr. Ehrenfeld: I am very much disturbed by the proposal that some patients with transient cerebral ischemic attacks will not be treated at all. I think we have come a long way since 1954, and we know a great deal more about this disease. One cannot take a patient who is having episodes of transient monocular blindness, or similar focal transient cerebral ischemic attacks and tell him you are not going to do anything.

The results from surgery have improved from all centers. Surely surgery is not perfect, but in the situation under consideration here the results are very good in terms of lowered morbidity and mortality and amelioration of symptoms. Perhaps aspirin is better, but I think it would be very unwise not to treat a patient at all.

Dr. Stallones: Dr. Dyken?

Dr. Dyken: Not being a member of your joint study, my only information is from what you publish. From the material published from this study, there seems to be for the first time some definite indications for surgery. In my experience in Indiana, a larger number of patients exists who do not answer the published criteria for surgery but still have atherosclerotic disease. It is either disseminated in multiple vessels, or it is not clear-cut. Therefore, I think a fairly large number of patients could be ethically treated with aspirin versus placebo. It is possible, and I think it is reasonable, and it could be worked out.

What we have been talking about is the design or construct of an experiment. This cannot be done in a conference such as this. It can be done only by the group that is going to be involved, the ones who are willing to become part of the study. A construct must be made so that it satisfies the investigators who are willing to undertake the study. They have to define the hypothesis. They have to survey the literature. They have to define a construct in terms that all participants can understand and agree upon. They must all use the same population and the same kind of treatment, etc. They cannot study all patients with cerebrovascular disease.

The participating group must define the population and treatment so that a completely alien group could repeat and verify the study. Verification is the basic one-word criterion for all biological experimentation. Therefore, those willing to participate must define a certain population, make a proper experimental design, and analyze the data and draw inferences from it. From this, they will have good information about one portion of the population.

Dr. Stallones: In view of the concern about the ethics of treating some people with aspirin and some people with placebo, one question which arises is related to how many of you are now treating your patients with aspirin? Is there a massive show of hands who are now using this therapy?

Dr. Dyken: You mean today or tomorrow?

Dr. Stallones: I was thinking about yesterday.

Dr. Dyken: Tomorrow I am starting.

Dr. Fields: Dr. Stallones asked Dr. McDowell whether or not he would agree to the post-operative treatment of his patients with aspirin. I feel sure that Dr. McDowell shares the view expressed to me several years ago by his late chief, Dr. Champ Lyons. Dr. Lyons stated, in no uncertain terms, that he felt that many of the published claims for long-term benefit from carotid endarterectomy were extravagant and not acceptable to him, because he was aware that most patients had intracranial atherosclerosis, as well as extracranial arterial disease. It seemed, therefore, more than a little ridiculous to him to make such extravagant claims as were being made by some of his colleagues in the field of vascular surgery.

Those of us who have been involved in the current study in which surgery has been a major focus are well aware of the advantage derived from an exchange of views between people from diverse backgrounds. We have come a long way in ten years toward defining the categories of patients who are candidates for a surgical operation. It has become obvious that the most suitable candidates are patients in whom there are clear-cut symptoms, defined as transient cerebral ischemic attacks, and in whom there is a lesion of greater than 50% stenosis in the cervical portion of the carotid artery. It is also evident that 90% of transient cerebral ischemic attacks in the carotid artery territory will cease after surgery, while 30% will cease spontaneously or 50% on medical treatment. There is certainly a difference between 30 or 50% and 90%.

Unfortunately, as I have already mentioned, we got locked into a specific definition of an obstructing lesion as one which produced a pressure gradient or a change in flow or could be considered as a significant stenosis. Then we were left with several questions. What is a "significant" stenosis? Is it radiographically significant? Is it clinically significant? Is it surgically significant? We must decide before we get into another study what is meant by the word "significant."

It is clear that surgery has a significant role in the management of cerebrovascular disease, and here I use the word "significant" to describe what has been accomplished in terms of surgical results.

When it is possible to reduce morbidity and mortality to less than 2% in the hands of experienced surgeons, we are talking about something feasible and reasonable, something that is truly significant.

The question which I believe is of particular concern to Dr. Wesley Moore of San Francisco, and his colleagues, is what to do about the type of patient who could not be admitted to the current study because he did not meet the criteria into which we were locked. If patients have radiographically demonstrated ulcerated lesions which are non-obstructing, can we justifiably allocate them into surgical and non-surgical treatment groups on a random basis?

If we randomly allocate surgical patients to treatment with aspirin or a placebo, post-operatively, we may have the opportunity to obtain a dividend. It is an accepted fact that the largest percent of deaths during follow-up is from myocardial infarction. It would be very interesting to learn whether or not the frequency of myocardial infarction could be reduced by treatment of post-surgical patients with aspirin. Dr. Weiss and his colleagues are very much interested in setting up a controlled clinical trial to determine whether aspirin is an efficacious agent in the prevention of myocardial infarction. He has kindly offered us his assistance in designing our study.

Dr. Stallones: Dr. Janeway, would you like to be heard?

Dr. Janeway: Dr. Hass, perhaps I did not make myself clear. I was not trying to look through either a telescope or a microscope. All I am saying is that we are not really talking about all transient cerebral ischemic attacks; we are talking about a particular type of transient cerebral ischemic attack. Why not define it as the transient cerebral ischemic attack due to fibrinoplatelet embolic phenomena. Unless you exclude all other things, or as many as you can, it is going to be difficult to arrive at an answer. I think Dr. McDowell and I agree that the more people you can cut out of the study, the easier it will be to arrive at an answer.

Dr. Stallones: Dr. Kricheff?

Dr. Kricheff: It seems to me, as I sit here and listen that your main problem is going to be the moral question. With the results in preventing transient cerebral ischemic attacks that our surgical colleagues have demonstrated, and the high incidence of occluded intracranial vessels that we have seen in the presence of irregularity and ulceration, it is going to be very difficult for the surgeons not to operate on those lesions which will be defined angiographically. This is a new ball game; the current cooperative study did not separate out the irregular or ulcerated plaques, and consequently, they were mixed in throughout the results.

The difference between using aspirin on patients and doing investigative surgery is reminiscent of the terminology used at the Pentagon, where the generals play war games with large computers. They talk about two types of decisions: One is a maximum probability decision, and the other is a minimum regret decision. These two things are very different. When you talk about surgery versus non-surgery, you want a maximum probability that the surgery will help the patient. On the other hand, when you use aspirin, which I think we will all agree has an exceedingly low morbidity and mortality, we are dealing with a minimum regret decision. The patient is interested primarily in a minimum regret decision; therefore, it is going to be very difficult, I would think, for the clinician who has responsibility for the patient not to put each and everyone on aspirin.

Dr. Stallones: I will ask Dr. Fields if he has any comments in closing this session.

Dr. Fields: All I have to say in closing is that I am very pleased that almost 100% of the persons who indicated they would attend were able to be here.

The material that has been put before us gives us much food for thought. It has been obvious from the discussions that any controlled clinical trial is going to take a great deal of careful planning. We will want to discuss this among those who are at least potential participants, and hopefully arrive at some tentative decisions which will enable us to develop a well-controlled study.

I hope that we can call on many who have attended this meeting, including those from the academic community and from the pharmaceutical industry, for advice and consultation in the development of a program.

INDEX